Critical Care in the Nursing Curriculum

Linking Education and Practice

Critical Care in the Nursing Curriculum

Linking Education and Practice

EDITORS

Barbara J. Daly, RN, MSN, CCRN, FAAN
Assistant Director of Nursing
University Hospital of Cleveland
Cleveland, Ohio

Jan Boller, RN, MSN
Manager of Program Development
American Association of Critical-Care Nurses
Newport Beach, California

AMERICAN ASSOCIATION OF CRITICAL-CARE NURSES
1990

AACN

Publications manager: Ellen French
Editorial consultant: Ramón Lavandero
Editorial assistants: Beth Wos
　　　　　　　　　　Kim Winchester
Copyeditor: Barbara Halliburton
Cover design: Donald P. Kibbe
Marketing: Ronald D. Carter
Typesetting, printing, binding: Port City Press

American Association of Critical-Care Nurses
P. O. Box 30008, Laguna Niguel, CA 92677

© 1990 by American Association of Critical-Care Nurses

All rights reserved. This book is protected by copyright. AACN authorizes individuals to photocopy items for internal or personal use. Other than individual use, no part of this book may be reproduced, stored in a retrieval system, or transmitted, in any form or by any means, electronic, mechanical, photocopying, recording, or otherwise, without prior written permission from AACN.

First edition published 1990
Printed in USA
93 92 91 90　　　5 4 3 2 1

ISBN 0-945812-07-8

proceedings from
AACN Invitational Conference

*Critical Care Nursing at the Baccalaureate Level
Strategies for the Future*

March 20-21, 1989
San Antonio, Texas

Contents

Preface / ix

Participants / xi

AACN Position Statements

   Integration of Critical Care Nursing Concepts and Clinical Experiences into Professional Nursing Programs / xxi

   Need for Critical Care Content and Clinical Experiences in Baccalaureate Nursing Curricula / xxiv

SECTION 1: Perspectives on Critical Care Content in Baccalaureate Curricula / 1

   Response to AACN Position Statements: The Education Perspective / 1
   Patty L. Hawken

   Response to AACN Position Statements: The Clinical Practice Perspective / 9
   Vernice Ferguson

   Response to Hawken and Ferguson: An Educator's Response / 15
   Sandra B. Dunbar

   Response to Hawken and Ferguson: A Clinical Manager's Response / 19
   Linda D. Searle

SECTION 2: Realities and Trends in Baccalaureate Education / 23

Performance Expectations of New Graduates / 23
Patricia Benner

Trends and Possibilities in Baccalaureate Nursing Programs / 41
Patricia Moccia

Response to Benner and Moccia: An Educator's Response / 52
Ellen B. Rudy

Response to Benner and Moccia: An Educator's Response / 59
Jeanette Lancaster

SECTION 3: Linking Education and Practice / 65

Relative Roles and Responsibilities of Education and Practice / 65
Sheila A. Ryan

Response to Ryan: An Educator's Perspective / 73
Clair E. Martin

Response to Ryan: A Nursing Administrator's Perspective / 78
Mary F. Woody

SECTION 4: Conclusion and Summaries / 83

Concluding Remarks / 83
Marguerite R. Kinney

Summary Reports from Triads / 85

Conference Summary / 90

SECTION 5: Appendixes / 95

A Survey of Critical Care Curriculum in Baccalaureate Programs in Nursing / 95

B *Critical Care Nursing in Baccalaureate Programs* / 101
Christine A. Tanner, Jeanette Hartshorn, Peri Rosenfeld

C *Getting Them Together* / 114
Molly Billingsley

Preface

In 1987, the American Association of Critical-Care Nurses (AACN) Board of Directors approved an implementation plan for the 1987 AACN position statement, *Need for Critical Care Content and Clinical Experience in Baccalaureate Nursing Curricula*. This position statement was based on AACN's concern with ensuring that academic education prepares nurses to care for today's critical care patient population.

The plan provided for an invitational conference with guest representatives from schools of nursing, hospitals, and professional nursing organizations. Nurses from large medical centers, small private hospitals, public and private schools, from across the United States were invited to respond to the position statement and recommend strategies for integrating critical care content into baccalaureate curricula. The conference was held March 20-21, 1989, in San Antonio, Texas.

In the same year, the Board of Directors also approved a proposal to work with the National League for Nursing (NLN) on a project to survey baccalaureate programs about the inclusion of critical care content in the programs' curricula (see Appendix A). A task force was appointed to plan the invitational conference and to work with NLN in a development of the survey.

This book describes the conference; the papers presented; the responses to the papers; and comments from triads of deans, nursing service administrators, and critical care educators. Conference recommendations to the Board of Directors of AACN and the results of the survey are included as *Critical Care Nursing in Baccalaureate Programs* (see Appendix B).

The Invitational Conference Task Force assumed that the major decisions about what is included in the baccalaureate curricula rest largely with faculty members, although these decisions clearly are influenced by the availability of clinical resources, faculty preparation, and external requirements, such as state board approval and NLN accreditation. Therefore, participants in the conference included groups or triads composed of faculty members involved in undergraduate education and curricular decision making, their deans, and counterparts in nursing service. Other participants were opinion leaders in nursing, involved in setting standards for state board examinations and NLN accreditation.

The purposes of the conference were as follows:

1. To examine issues surrounding the inclusion of critical care nursing content in the baccalaureate curriculum.
2. To achieve consensus on the need to integrate critical care nursing content into the baccalaureate curriculum.
3. To achieve consensus on the education of nurses who care for critically ill patients.
4. To develop recommendations and strategies regarding the educational preparation of nurses in critical care nursing.

Influential nursing leaders, knowledgeable about education and practice in critical care nursing, prepared and distributed papers, in advance of the conference, on issues related to critical care nursing in the baccalaureate curriculum. At the conference, they presented summaries of their papers. The papers were followed by responses in which two or more perspectives on the issues were presented and debated. Small groups were then convened to discuss the issues identified in the papers, seek a consensus on the issues, and develop strategies to address them. Issues addressed in these discussions included attitudes and beliefs about critical care nursing content in the baccalaureate curriculum, trends in baccalaureate education, the knowledge and skills needed at graduation for care of patients with life-threatening conditions, and the relative roles of the nursing service and nursing education in the teaching of critical care nursing.

Edited transcripts of the papers and panel discussions are presented. Summaries of the responses to a questionnaire distributed at the end of the conference are also provided. Finally, a summary of AACN's response to the conference is provided, outlining strategies for the future to promote basic education for nurses who care for critically ill patients.

Participants

AACN Invitational Conference
*Critical Care Nursing at the Baccalaureate Level
Strategies for the Future*
March 20-21, 1989
San Antonio, Texas

Conference Planning Task Force

Christine Tanner, RN, PhD, FAAN, Professor, School of Nursing, Oregon Health Sciences University, Portland, Oregon

Kathleen J. Andreoli, RN, DSN, Dean and Vice President, Rush University Presbyterian-St. Luke's Medical Center, Chicago, Illinois

Jan Boller, RN, MSN, Manager of Program Development, American Association of Critical-Care Nurses, Newport Beach, California

Bonnie Chenevey, RN, MS, Director of Certification, AACN Certification Corporation, Newport Beach, California

Barbara Daly, RN, MSN, CCRN, FAAN, Assistant Director of Nursing, University Hospital of Cleveland, Cleveland, Ohio

Sandra K. Goodnough, RN, MSN, Board Member, American Association of Critical-Care Nurses, Doctoral Student, Texas Woman's University, Houston, Texas

Marguerite R. Kinney, RN, DNSc, FAAN, Past President, AACN, Editor, *Focus on Critical Care*, Professor of Nursing, University of Alabama at Birmingham, Birmingham, Alabama

Presenters

Patricia Benner, RN, PhD, FAAN, Associate Professor, Department of Physiological Nursing, University of California, San Francisco, San Francisco, California

Sandra B. Dunbar, RN, DSN, Past President, AACN, Associate Professor and, Coordinator of Critical Care Nursing, Nell Hodgson Woodruff School of Nursing, Emory University, Atlanta, Georgia

Vernice Ferguson, RN, MA, FAAN, FRCN, Deputy Assistant Chief Medical Director, of Nursing Programs, The Veterans Administration, Washington, District of Columbia

Patty L. Hawken, RN, PhD, Dean and Professor, School of Nursing, The University of Texas Health Science Center, at San Antonio, San Antonio, Texas

Jeanette Lancaster, RN, PhD, FAAN, Dean and Professor, School of Nursing, Wright State University-Miami Valley, Dayton, Ohio

Clair E. Martin, RN, PhD, Dean and Professor, Nell Hodgson Woodruff School of Nursing, Emory University, Atlanta, Georgia

Patricia Moccia, RN, PhD, Vice President, Division of Education and Accreditation Services, National League for Nursing, New York, New York

Ellen B. Rudy, RN, PhD, FAAN, Chairperson, Edward J. and Louise Mellon, Professor of Acute Care Nursing, Case Western Reserve University, Cleveland, Ohio

Sheila A. Ryan, PhD, RN, FAAN, Dean and Director, Medical Center Nursing, University of Rochester, Rochester, New York

Linda D. Searle, RN, MN, CNA, Past President, AACN, Clinical Nursing Director, Surgical Nursing Department, Cedar-Sinai Medical Center, Los Angeles, California

Mary F. Woody, RN, MA, FAAN, Associate Hospital Director, Director of Nursing, Emory University Hospital, Atlanta, Georgia

Guests

Jo Eleanor Elliott, RN, FAAN, Director, Division of Nursing, Bureau of Health Professions, U.S. Public Health Service, Rockville, Maryland

Renatta Loquist, RN, MN, President, National Council of State Boards of Nursing, Executive Director, South Carolina Board of Nursing, Columbia, South Carolina

Robert V. Piemonte, EdD, RN, CAE, FAAN, Executive Director, National Student Nurses' Association, New York, New York

Small Group Leaders

Kathleen Burke, RN, MSN, CCRN, Lecturer, School of Nursing, University of Pennsylvania, Philadelphia, Pennsylvania

Kathleen J. Andreoli, RN, DSN, Dean and Vice President, Rush Presbyterian-St. Luke's Medical Center, Chicago, Illinois

Diane Billings, RN, EdD, Professor of Nursing and Baccalaureate Program, Curriculum Coordinator-Evaluator, Indiana University School of Nursing, Indianapolis, Indiana

Jan M. H. Brewer, RN, PhD, Director of Professional Development, American Association of Critical-Care Nurses, Newport Beach, California

Margaret Bruya, RN, DNSc, Associate Professor, Intercollegiate Center for Nursing Education, Spokane, Washington

Barbara Daly, RN, MSN, CCRN, FAAN, Assistant Director of Nursing and, Assistant Clinical Professor, University Hospitals of Cleveland and, Case Western Reserve University, Cleveland, Ohio

Sandra B. Dunbar, RN, DSN, Past President, American Association of Critical-Care Nurses, Associate Professor & Coordinator of Critical Care Nursing, Nell Hodgson Woodruff School of Nursing, Emory University, Atlanta, Georgia

Sandra K. Goodnough, RN, MSN, Board Member, American Association of Critical-Care Nurses, Doctoral Student, Texas Woman's University, Houston, Texas

Joanne M. Krumberger, RN, MSN, CCRN, Critical Care Clinical Nurse Specialist, Milwaukee VA Medical Center, Milwaukee, Wisconsin

Linda F. Samson, PhD, RNC, Board Member, American Association of Critical-Care Nurses, Assistant Professor of Nursing, Kennesaw State College, Marietta, Georgia

Karen Sechrist, RN, PhD, Director of Research, American Association of Critical-Care Nurses, Newport Beach, California

Madeline Wake, RN, PhD, Assistant Professor of Nursing, Marquette University, Milwaukee, Wisconsin

TRIADS: DEAN/FACULTY/CLINICAL ADMINISTRATOR

Region I (North Atlantic): *Connecticut, Delaware, District of Columbia, Maine, Massachusetts, New Hampshire, New Jersey, New York, Pennsylvania, Rhode Island, Vermont*

Albright College, Reading, Pennsylvania

Barbara Haus, RN, EdD, Chairperson, Department of Nursing

Gloria Miller, RN, MSN, Vice President, Nursing, Reading Hospital and Medical Center

Catholic University of America, Washington, District of Columbia

Lois Hoskins, RN, PhD, Dean, School of Nursing

Colleen Norton, RN, MSN, CCRN, Assistant Professor

Helen Bowles, RN, MSN, Instructor, Professional Development & Nursing Marketing, Washington Hospital Center

Massachusetts General Hospital, Boston, Massachusetts

Elizabeth M. Grady, RN, PhD, Professor and Director Graduate Program in Nursing, MGH Institute of Health Professions

Joan B. Fitzmaurice, RN, PhD, Director, Quality Assurance and Research

Yvonne Munn, RN, MSN, Associate General Director, Director of Nursing

Syracuse University, Syracuse, New York

Cecilia Mulvey, RN, PhD, Associate Dean for Academic Affairs, College of Nursing

Ann Sedore, RN, PhD, Associate Professor, College of Nursing

University of Pennsylvania, Philadelphia, Pennsylvania

Mary D. Naylor, RN, PhD, FAAN, Associate Dean and Director of Undergraduate Studies, School of Nursing

Joanne Disch, RN, PhD, Past President, AACN, Clinical Director of Medical Nursing, Hospital of the University of Pennsylvania

Kathleen McCauley, RN, MSN, CS, Cardiovascular Clinical Specialist, Hospital of the University of Pennsylvania

University of Rhode Island, Kingston, Rhode Island

Jean R. Miller, PhD, RN, Dean, College of Nursing

Jacqueline Fortin, RN, DNSc, Associate Professor, College of Nursing

Suzanne Sawtelle, RN, BSN, CCRN, Clinical Educator, Rhode Island Hospital

Villanova University, Villanova, Pennsylvania

Marita Frain, RN, EdM, Director of Undergraduate Program, School of Nursing

Margaret Kendrick, RN, MSN, Assistant Professor of Nursing

Ann Stolarik, MSN, CCRN, Clinical Nurse Educator, Bryn Mawr Hospital

Yale University, New Haven, Connecticut

Judith B. Krauss, RN, MSN, Dean and Professor, School of Nursing

Mairead Hickey, RN, PhD (c), Assistant Professor and Coordinator,, Cardiovascular Nursing, School of Nursing

Laura Mylott, RN, MSN, Clinical Nurse Specialist, Cardiac Surgery, Yale-New Haven Hospital

> **Region II** (Midwest): *Illinois, Indiana, Iowa, Kansas, Michigan, Minnesota, Missouri, Nebraska, North Dakota, Ohio, South Dakota, Wisconsin*

Creighton University, Omaha, Nebraska

Shirley Dooling, RN, EdD, Dean, School of Nursing

Anita Larsen, RN, CCRN, Nurse Manager, Critical Care Services, St. Joseph Hospital

Jackie Thielen, RN, MSN, CCRN, Critical Care Clinical Specialist, Methodist Hospital

Kent State University, Kent, Ohio

P. Joan Dashield, RN, MSN, Associate Professor, School of Nursing

Carol Pankratz, RN, MSN, Adjunct Instructor, Staff Development, Akron General Medical Center

Marquette University, Milwaukee, Wisconsin

Ardene Brown, RN, PhD, Associate Dean for Academic Affairs, College of Nursing

Darlene Weis, PhD, Assistant Professor, College of Nursing

Mennonite College, Bloomington, Illinois

Kathleen A. Hogan, PhD, Vice President/Dean, College of Nursing

Rebecca R. Sutter, RN, MN, CNS, Associate Professor of Medical-Surgical Nursing, Clinical Nurse Specialist

Marilyn Travers, RN, Director, Critical Care, Brokaw Hospital

The Ohio State University, Columbus, Ohio

Carol F. Baker, RN, PhD, Assistant Professor, Department of Life Span Process, College of Nursing

Linda K. Daley, RN, MS, Instructor of Life Span Process, College of Nursing

Susan Alden, RN, MS, Director of Critical Care and Oncology Nursing, The Ohio State University Hospital

South Dakota State University, Brookings, South Dakota

Carmen Westwick, RN, PhD, Dean, College of Nursing

Pamela A. Schroeder, RN, MEd, MS, Assistant Professor, College of Nursing

Martha Iken, RN, MS, Critical Care Float Nurse/Education Services, Sioux Valley Hospital, Sioux Falls, South Dakota

University of Michigan, Ann Arbor, Michigan

Elisabeth Pennington, RN, EdD, Assistant Dean, Undergraduate Studies, School of Nursing

Patricia M. Butler, RN, PhD, Assistant Professor of Nursing

Joan O. Robinson, RN, MS, Interim Associate Hospital Administrator and Director of Nursing, University of Michigan Medical Center

Region III (Southern): *Alabama, Arkansas, Florida, Georgia, Kentucky, Louisiana, Maryland, Mississippi, North Carolina, Oklahoma, South Carolina, Tennessee, Texas, Virginia, West Virginia*

George Mason University, Fairfax, Virginia

Rita M. Carty, RN, DNSc, FAAN, Dean, School of Nursing

E. Francine Roberts, RN, MSN, Assistant Clinical Professor

Mary Jane Mastrovich, RN, MSN, Associate Director of Nursing, Fairfax Hospital

Nell Hodgson Woodruff School of Nursing, Emory University, Atlanta, Georgia

Clair E. Martin, RN, PhD, Dean and Professor, Nell Hodgson Woodruff School of Nursing

Margaret Parsons, RN, PhD, Chair and Professor, Adult Health Division

Mary F. Woody RN, MA, FAAN, Associate Hospital Director, Director of Nursing, Emory University Hospital

Texas Christian University, Fort Worth, Texas

Patricia Scearse, RN, DNSc, Dean, Harris College of Nursing

Alice Gaul, RN, PhD, Assistant Professor

Jamie Bankston, RN, Harris Hospital Methodist

University of Florida, Gainesville, Florida

Lois Malasanos, RN, PhD, Dean and Professor, College of Nursing

Gloria Chiras, RN, MSN, Assistant Professor, College of Nursing

Myrna Courage, RN, PhD, Director, Junior Studies, College of Nursing

Betty Jermier, RN, MSN, Program Director - Orientation, Shands Hospital

University of Kentucky, Lexington, Kentucky

Mary Walker, RN, PhD, Chair and Associate Professor, Division of Adult Nursing, College of Nursing

Pamela Kidd, RN, CEN, PhD (c), Assistant Professor, College of Nursing

Linda M. Holtzclaw, RN, MSN, Staff Development Instructor, University of Kentucky Medical Center

University of Maryland, Baltimore, Maryland

Nan Hechenberger, PhD, Dean and Professor, University of Maryland School of Nursing

Robert Ismeurt, RN, PhD, Assistant Professor, School of Nursing

Lynn Gerber Smith, RN, MS, Nursing Education Coordinator, Maryland Institute for Emergency Medical Services Systems

University of North Carolina, at Chapel Hill, Chapel Hill, North Carolina

Eleanor Browning, MSN, Associate Professor, Director Undergraduate Studies, School of Nursing

Barbara Bunker, RN, MSN, Associate Professor

Chris Winkelman, RNC, MSN, CCRN, Clinical Nurse Supervisor, North Carolina Memorial Hospital

The University of Texas, Austin, Austin, Texas

LaVerne Gallman, PhD, Professor and Interim Dean, School of Nursing

Sarah Peters, RN, MSN, Instructor of Clinical Nursing

Donna Huckabee, RN, CCRN, Head Nurse, ICU-CCU, Brackenridge Hospital

> **Region IV** (Western): *Alaska, Arizona, California, Colorado, Hawaii, Idaho, Montana, Nevada, New Mexico, Oregon, Utah, Washington, Wyoming*

Arizona State University, Tempe, Arizona

Barbara K. Miller, PhD, Associate Professor and Chair, Adult/Health Medical-Surgical Division, College of Nursing

Shirley Bell, RN, MSN, EdD, Assistant Professor, College of Nursing

Marjorie Hill, RN, MS, CCRN, Adjunct Faculty - Clinical Instructor, Desert Samaritan Hospital, Arizona State University College of Nursing

Brigham Young University, Provo, Utah

Donna Boland, RN, PhD, Associate Dean, College of Nursing

Renea Lindstrom, RN, MS, CCRN, Instructor, School of Nursing

Judy Blaufuss, RN, MS, Director of Critical Care Nursing, Latter Day Saints Hospital, Salt Lake City, Utah

California State University, Los Angeles, Los Angeles, California

Jo Ann Johnson, RN, DPA, Department Chair, School of Nursing

Christine Latham, RN, MSN, CCRN, Associate Professor, School of Nursing

Ann Kaiser, RN, BA, Associate Administrator, Huntington Memorial Hospital, Pasadena, California

Intercollegiate Center for Nursing Education, Spokane, Washington

Lorna Schumann, RN, PhD, CCRN, ARNP, Assistant Professor

Karen Groth, RN, MN, CS, Instructor

Montana State University, Bozeman, Montana

Kathleen A. Long, RN, PhD, CS, FAAN, Assistant Dean and Associate Professor, College of Nursing

Vonna Koehler, RN, MN, Assistant Professor, College of Nursing

Sharon Dieziger, RN, BSN, Director, Critical Care, Montana Deaconess Medical Center, Great Falls, Montana

University of California, Los Angeles, Los Angeles, California

Ada Lindsey, RN, PhD, FAAN, Dean and Professor, School of Nursing

Gen Bahu, RN, Lecturer, UCLA School of Nursing

Suzette Cardin, RN, MSN, CCRN, Nurse Manager, CCU/COU, UCLA Medical Center

University of California, San Francisco, San Francisco, California

Marilyn E. Flood, RN, PhD, Associate Dean, Academic Programs, School of Nursing

Phylita Skov, RN, MS, Assistant Clinical Professor, Department of Physiological Nursing

Maura A. Hopkins, RN, MSN, Nurse Manager, Intensive Care Unit, University of California, San Francisco Medical Center

University of Northern Colorado, Greeley, Colorado

Sandy Baird, RN, EdD, Assistant Director, School of Nursing

Jane Koeckeritz, RN, MS, Assistant Professor, School of Nursing

Patricia Wilson, RN, MS, Nursing Care Coordinator, CCU, North Colorado Medical Center

University of Washington, Seattle, Washington

Joan Shaver, RN, PhD, Chair and Associate Professor, Department of Physiological Nursing

Sharon Fought, RN, PhD, Assistant Professor, School of Nursing

Janet Marvin, RN, MN, Associate Professor, School of Nursing, Associate Director, Burn Center, Harborview Medical Center

AACN POSITION STATEMENT

Integration of Critical Care Nursing Concepts and Clinical Experiences into Professional Nursing Programs*

WHEREAS, the philosophy of the American Association of Critical-Care Nurses is that each critically ill person has the right to expect nursing care provided by a critical care nurse, and

WHEREAS, AACN has accepted the American Nurses Association (ANA) definition of nursing as "the diagnosis and treatment of human responses to actual or potential health problems" and has defined critical care nursing as that specialty within nursing which deals specifically with human responses to life-threatening problems; and

WHEREAS, critical care nursing practice is the utilization of the nursing process in the prevention of and intervention in life-threatening situations, and

WHEREAS, the scope of critical care nursing practice is dynamic and includes any environment in which the critically ill patient is found, and

WHEREAS, integral components of critical care nursing practice include individual accountability and lifelong learning, and

WHEREAS, caring for the critically ill patient provides the professional nursing student with an opportunity to develop

---

*See also AACN position statement, *Need for Critical Care Content and Clinical Experiences in Baccalaureate Nursing Curricula.*

a) a thorough knowledge of the interrelatedness of body systems and the dynamic nature of the life process,

b) a recognition and appreciation of the individual's wholeness, uniqueness and significant social and environmental relationships, and

c) an appreciation of the importance of the collaborative role of all members of the health care team; then

BE IT RESOLVED THAT,

1. The American Association of Critical-Care Nurses recognize that the use of the nursing process is essential to the planning, implementation and evaluation of education in critical care nursing.

2. Students operationalize, in consultation with faculty and critical care practitioners, the nursing process with critically ill persons and their families by

   a) collecting subjective and objective data to determine needs,b) making assessments based upon data collected,
   c) formulating nursing diagnoses,
   d) planning appropriate interventions,
   e) coordinating the appropriate care for specific interventions given by other health team members,
   f) implementing the plan of care according to priority of needs and own levels of ability,
   g) evaluating care given, revising as necessary,

AND students routinely evaluate their own learning needs, plan appropriate methods of meeting these needs and continue this self-evaluation process after entry into licensed nursing practice.

3. Nursing faculty present concepts at a level appropriate for students' educational levels and select clinical experiences with patients at an acuity level appropriate to students' capabilities.

BE IT FURTHER RESOLVED THAT,
Nursing faculty consult with nursing staff of critical care areas in order to plan meaningful learning experiences for students.

Primary responsibility for student supervision resides with the nursing faculty; however, critical care practitioners shall retain patient care accountability.

Nursing faculty and critical care practitioners jointly maintain appropriate supervision of students so that bedside practice standards are maintained.

Those who supervise nursing students shall

- a) have a recommended minimum of a baccalaureate degree in nursing for critical care nurse practitioners, or a graduate degree appropriate for nursing faculty;
- b) demonstrate current clinical expertise in critical care nursing;
- c) demonstrate application of knowledge of current critical care nursing literature; and
- d) demonstrate application of theoretical knowledge in the clinical supervision of professional nursing students.

Adopted by AACN Board of Directors, November 1983 (amended July 1984).

AACN POSITION STATEMENT

Need For Critical Care Content and Clinical Experiences in Baccalaureate Nursing Curricula*

BACCALAUREATE NURSING PROGRAMS are responsible for providing graduates with the requisite skills to render nursing care to society. In order to accomplish this goal, nursing educators must continuously assure that their curricula are reflective of society's needs. The rapidly occurring changes in society and the health care system require nursing education programs to re-evaluate and revise their current curricula to ensure that graduates are prepared to meet society's health care needs.

WHEREAS, there are increasing levels of acuity and complexity of patient problems in most health care settings, and

WHEREAS, there are increasing numbers of patients in most health care settings who are physiologically supported by advanced medical therapeutics and technology previously reserved for use only in critical care settings, and

WHEREAS, there is an increase in the number of elderly in society who have acute and chronic complex illnesses, and

WHEREAS, there are fiscal constraint effecting the health care industry which result in patient's early discharge from hospital to home or community health agencies, and

---

*See also AACN position statement, *Integration of Critical Care Nursing Concepts and Clinical Experiences into Professional Nursing Programs.*

WHEREAS, there are selected concepts traditionally thought to be solely within the domain of critical care nursing practice which are now applicable to many other areas of nursing practice, and

WHEREAS, there is a necessity for professional nurses in most health care settings to apply critical care knowledge and skills to patient care, and

WHEREAS, there is a need to provide professional nursing students with the knowledge and skills to practice at an entry level in the care of patients with complex problems and needs, and

WHEREAS, there are unique clinical experiences in the critical care environment which provide professional nursing students with the opportunity to acquire the knowledge and skills to practice at an entry level in the care of patients with complex problems and needs;

THEREFORE, BE IT HEREBY RESOLVED THAT, AACN strongly recommends incorporation of critical care content and corresponding direct clinical experiences into baccalaureate nursing programs; and

BE IT FURTHER RESOLVED THAT, AACN strongly recommends, in conjunction with baccalaureate schools of nursing and appropriate accrediting bodies, of the development, implementation and evaluation of strategies to incorporate critical care content and direct clinical experiences in baccalaureate nursing curricula; and

BE IT FURTHER RESOLVED THAT, AACN strongly urges nursing administrators and educators to develop mechanisms to facilitate direct clinical experiences for students with critically ill patients.

References

AACN, *Integration of Critical Care Nursing Concepts and Clinical Experiences into Professional Nursing Programs,* AACN Position Statement, July, 1984.

AACN, *Education Standards for Critical Care Nursing.* St. Louis: The C. V. Mosby Company, 1986.

AACN, *Standards for Nursing Care of the Critically Ill,* Reston, VA, Reston Publishing Company, 1981.

Andreoli, K. G., & Musser, L. A., Trends That May Affect Nursing's Future, *Nursing & Health Care,* January 1985, Vol 6, No. 1, p.47.

Dunbar, S., Imperatives for Nursing Education, *Heart & Lung,* Vol. 15, No. 6, November 1986.

Levine, E., Hospital Headlines, *Hospitals,* 54:18-19, 1980.

Adopted by AACN Board of Directors, February 1987.

SECTION 1
Perspectives on Critical Care Content in Baccalaureate Curricula

Response to AACN Position Statements: The Education Perspective

Patty L. Hawken

The efforts by the AACN (1984, 1987) to develop and publish a position statement on the need for critical care content and experiences in a baccalaureate nursing program are commendable and should be explored carefully. Since 1983, with the start of the prospective payment system for Medicare patients and the development of the diagnosis related groups, the patients admitted to and staying in hospitals are those who are in an acute phase of their illness. Diagnostic tests are being done before hospitalization, and total recovery and rehabilitation have been shifted to homes, clinics, and the community. Nurses working in hospitals are caring for patients in the most vulnerable time of the patients' illness. Since 68% of all employed nurses work in hospitals, it is imperative that all students enrolled and subsequently graduating from baccalaureate programs have a clear understanding of critical care nursing. Further, they should have the requisite skills and decision-making ability to care for patients in a compassionate, intelligent manner.

A recent summary analysis (Levine & Associates, 1988) of critical care done for AACN by Levine and Associates indicated that there are 223,000 critical care nurses, and yet the need projected for 1990 will be in the range of 300,000 to 365,000. This is a 40% to 65% increase in the number of nurses who need to be attracted to critical care nursing in a short time. The question is truly whether the service sector and educational institutions can meet this demand.

As an educator, I strongly believe that the education of a student in nursing should reflect the reality of society, society's trends, future directions, and perceived needs. One of the responsibilities of nurse educators is to anticipate and recognize societal changes and needs and to ensure that nursing curricula are responsive to these identified needs. Another responsibility is to eliminate content areas or foci that have lost relevance or become less important in the larger scheme of things. Changes in curricula occur as a result of faculty members within schools of nursing determining the content, clinical experiences, and outcome abilities for students. The question then comes down to: How does a specialty group influence the faculty members of schools of nursing to consider content and clinical experiences in the area of the specialty group? To influence any group, it is necessary first to know something about the group's members. It is also necessary to know strategies to influence others, and certainly, to have a good product. The flip side of the coin is to avoid strategies that will detract from a position: championing, demanding, threatening, overpowering, and so forth. Strategies are mentioned because educators are inundated with specialty groups and others championing for their specialty, cause, or area of content and literally demanding more curriculum time. Today, we are being pressured to include more time for ethical issues, legal concerns, cultural connotations, health policy, computer applications, home care, elder care, emergency department care, operating room care, to name a few of the content areas.

Defining Critical Care

In considering the factors necessary to influence a group, let me start with the product, or in this case, content area. As I read the *Need for Critical Care Content and Clinical Experiences in Baccalaureate Nursing Curricula* (AACN, 1987), I initially could support the resolves and resolutions. The overall concept, in other words, seems obvious, and needed, something schools of nursing should strive for. As I began to study the document, however, I became confused. I was looking for a definition of critical care and what specifically was needed in the curriculum according to AACN. I saw "levels of acuity," "complex patient problems," "unique clinical experiences", and "critically ill patients" used throughout the document, and I began to ask myself, What is critical care? Does critical care encompass a concept, population, group of services, or environment? What is the role, scope, and focus of critical care? Before, I always had thought of critical care as a concept: a facet of nursing that encompassed care of a patient who had a life-threatening condition. The patient could be any age, and the life-threatening condition was a present condition, not an anticipated or potential one. Perhaps my idea of critical care was too narrow.

I decided to go to the literature and find out from the critical care textbooks what critical care nursing really is. Here are some of my findings. Kinney, Packa, & Dunbar, 1988, p. 4), defined critical care as "that specialty within nursing which deals with human responses to life-threatening problems." Does critical care include patients threatening suicide, patients who are severely obese, or patients who have anorexia nervosa or alcoholism? I never had categorized these human responses as critical care concerns, but maybe they are.

Kinney et al. (1988, p.4) went on to say that "critical care is goal directed, and endeavors to ensure effective interaction of three requisites — the patient, nurse, and environment. Critical care has a framework within which it is practiced based on a body of knowledge and application of that knowledge through the nursing process." Is not all of this true for any specialty within nursing? If community health, pediatrics, or maternity were substituted for critical care, would not the sentence still be true? I was becoming more confused. Does critical care refer to care of patients in acute situations in maternity, pediatric, psychiatric situations? Again I had compartmentalized the critical care nurse as one who cares for the adult patient who has a medical or surgical problem.

Hudak, Gallo, & Lohr, (1986, p.3) stated "Essence of critical care nursing lies not in special environments or amid special equipment but in the nurse's decision-making process and willingness to act on decisions made." Could this not be said of any nurse in any specialty? Substitute the name of another specialty, and the revised statement would be endorsed by that specialty group.

The intent is not to critique textbooks, but I reviewed four major texts (Holloway, 1988; Hudak et al, 1986; Kenner et al., 1985; & Kinney et al., 1988) on critical care nursing, and regardless of their focus, they were not able to differentiate clearly critical care nursing from other specialties. Some books referred to the holistic process, and all used the nursing process. There is nothing wrong with any of this. I substituted the word nursing without a modifier, and most of the definitions were good definitions of nursing.

One of the best indicators of critical care was presented in the *Sixth Report to the President and Congress on the Status of Health Personnel in the United States*, (U.S. Department of Health and Human Services, 1988). In the nursing section, the panel differentiated critical care from acute or complex care, placing critical care as the most specialized and indicating that "critical care encompassed all patients whose conditions were totally unstable, totally nursing dependent, requiring sophisticated technologies and thus requiring many hours of care per patient day" (p. 10-64). Patients with acute or complex problems were defined as "totally nursing care dependent, medically unstable, and labile and frequently dependent upon sophisticated technologies. They may be in life-threatening situations or in end stages of disease but would need fewer hours of care than critical care patients" (p. 10-64). These definitions are closer to my concept of critical care nursing.

My basic concern is that AACN needs to define critical care clearly, to the extent that critical care is defined by what it is and what it is not. Does critical care encompass care of children? Does critical care nursing really encompass potential threats to life (e.g., severe obesity, drugs, alcoholism), or is the focus on the care of the adult patient who is experiencing a life threatening crisis? This is the first step: being clear and consistent about what is perceived to be the specialty and then articulating this definition. Help in this area may be found in the article by Reed & Hoffman (1986), "The Enigma of Graduate Nursing Education: Advanced Generalist? Specialist?". The article outlines a paradigm for organizing graduate education; yet it could be applied to both graduate and undergraduate areas. The three areas stressed are focus, scope, and depth. These three areas need to be addressed in relation to critical care, and this will also help differentiate undergraduate emphasis from graduate specialty.

Another help might be to review other specialty areas' guides as a model. The pamphlet on cultural diversity in the nursing curriculum by the American Nurses' Association (ANA 1986) outlines purposes and objectives, strategies for developing philosophy and goals of the curriculum. The guide also outlines a concept approach, a unit approach, and a course approach to this content area. This document is clear and inclusive and helps educators see what the product is — in this case, content that should be included in the curriculum.

AACN Recommendations

Once we have a clear definition of critical care — what it is and what it is not — AACN then needs to define content that is imperative for a baccalaureate student and to differentiate this content from 1990 programs in graduate study. Each of the resolutions in AACN's position statement needs to be expanded to help faculty members understand the intent and direction.

First, AACN strongly recommends "incorporation of critical care content and corresponding direct clinical experiences into baccalaureate nursing programs" (AACN, 1987). This could be expanded by saying, "as defined by AACN document X." Then document X should define content that is considered critical care content. Or if specific content cannot be teased out, examples should be given of situations that would be specific for the critical care nurse with a baccalaureate degree to handle expertly. The importance of defining the content cannot be understated. If AACN wants to be effective in moving nursing forward, it needs to communicate the message clearly. Once a decision is made about content, then it will be easier to identify direct clinical experiences. Finding patients to care for who demonstrate or illustrate the content will be simplified, and this will give specific direction to faculty members.

"Into baccalaureate nursing programs", is an important notion. I agree with this notion. However, the facts are that approximately 61% of all nurses in critical care areas in hospitals have associate degrees or diplomas. It is clear that AACN is urging that this content be placed in baccalaureate programs. Does AACN want to encourage or discourage critical care content in associate degree and diploma programs or remain silent on this issue? Does AACN want to differentiate content appropriate for associate degree and diploma programs from baccalaureate education? The issue is today's reality (nurses with associate degrees are prepared to do some critical care and are put in these positions) vs. a goal to be achieved (enough baccalaureate nurses prepared to be exclusively critical care nurses). Perhaps a conscious decision was made to exclude associate degree and diploma programs. If so, that is the association's prerogative. If, however, it just was not addressed, then I think it needs to be addressed so that the position of AACN is clear. The present numbers of needed critical care nurses and the future projections indicate that for several years to come, we will rely on various levels of educational preparation in critical care.

Second, AACN strongly recommends "in conjunction with baccalaureate schools of nursing and appropriate accrediting bodies, the development, implementation and evaluation of strategies to incorporate critical care content and direct clinical experiences in baccalaureate nursing curricula," (AACN, 1987). "In conjunction with" are the important three words. The critical care specialist needs to be involved intimately in curriculum development, and this can be done only if individuals with critical care expertise, who are caring for patients on a daily basis, join with the faculty members who are preparing classes and teaching students. Cooperation and collaboration are essential and, in fact, are the key to facilitating changes in nursing curricula.

Let me mention accrediting bodies. Schools of nursing are accredited by state boards, regional accrediting agencies and specialty accrediting organizations, (in our case, through the NLN). Agency members of the NLN Council of Baccalaureate and Higher Degree Program (1988) decide the criteria for accreditation. The criteria do not include specific content areas. The council carefully has avoided any criterion that would designate an area of content because nursing is dynamic and the criteria need to reflect the school and the parent institution. One example of a criterion of the NLN is that the "curriculum provides theoretical and clinical learning activities in health promotion and maintenance, illness care and rehabilitation of clients" (Council of Baccalaureate and Higher Degree Programs, 1988, p.7). This is as close to a specific area of content as an accrediting group will come. So eliminating the words "and appropriate accrediting bodies" seems to me to be acceptable without changing intent. Working with faculty members is the important ingredient.

Third, AACN strongly urges "nursing administrators and educators to develop mechanisms to facilitate direct clinical experiences for students with critical patients" (AACN, 1987). All schools of nursing have mechanisms in place to negotiate their present clinical experiences. If AACN is expressing concern that some agencies do not allow students experience with critically ill patients, then this needs to be worked out with the school of nursing administrators and the particular agency. Perhaps using preceptors from the hospital to work with students on a one-to-one basis in the care of the critically ill is a way to provide students this experience and exposure. This type of negotiation would follow the development and agreement by faculty in relation to the nature of the content and clinical experience to demonstrate that content.

Strategies

Next strategies need to be developed to communicate critical care content to faculty members. One of the ways AACN can tell its story and convince faculty members to make curriculum changes would be to take the message to the faculty. At the November 1988 meeting of the Council of Baccalaureate and Higher Degree Programs, Jeanette Hartshorn, past president of AACN, served on a panel to discuss critical care in the curriculum, along with two additional persons, one to discuss gerontology and another to discuss home care. Faculty members had the opportunity to hear these presentations and to carry the message back to their own schools. The message needs to be clear in relation to critical care and should include a definition, description, and outline of content that would be appropriate.

Another strategy already mentioned would be for AACN to do its own publication similar to the ANA's cultural diversity document, the gerontological nursing document, and others that have a specialty area to describe and highlight. This document could then be shared with faculty throughout the United States, with the notion that some consistency in relation to the discipline would be communicated. A third strategy would be to have each critical care nurse in AACN contact faculty members personally at schools in the nurse's area and ask to meet with the curriculum committee and present a case for critical care content. Also, critical care nurses in the community should be volunteering to serve on school of nursing committees so their input would be heard. Critical care nurses who are faculty members have a key role to play within their faculty and need to discuss the issue and move forward with curriculum changes. A fourth strategy is to publish articles in journals read by nurse educators. Not all faculty members read critical care journals, and you may end up preaching to the choir if publishing your concerns and solutions is done only in your own specialty journals.

These are just a few strategies to think about in relation to the intent of the position statement. As my charge was to critique the position statement, not write one, I obviously have the easy task. To summarize my critique, the idea that generated the position is a good one: that preparation in critical care nursing needs to be included in all baccalaureate programs. The specifics need to be developed in detail, so answers to questions such as what is critical care nursing, how does it differ from nursing in general and from other specialties in particular, and what content is essential can be answered and agreed by all. Then strategies need to be developed to take this message to faculty members collectively and individually. Once a case is made with a good plan in place, the chances of having this position adopted by faculty groups are good. I urge the AACN to move forward with vigor and enthusiasm. Your direction is needed and wanted, and many are waiting for the specifics.

References

American Association of Critical-Care Nurses.(1984). *Integration of critical care nursing concepts and clinical experiences into professional nursing programs* (AACN position statement). Newport Beach, CA: Author.

American Association of Critical-Care Nurses.(1987). *Need for critical care content and clinical experiences in baccalaureate nursing curricula.*(AACN position statement). Newport Beach, CA: Author.

American Association of Critical-Care Nurses. (1988). *Summary analysis of critical care nurse supply and requirements.* Newport Beach, CA: Author.

American Nurses' Association. (1986). *Cultural diversity in the nursing curriculum: A guide for implementation.* Kansas City, MO: Author.

Council of Baccalaureate and Higher Degree Programs.(1988). *Criteria for the evaluation of baccalaureate and higher degree programs in nursing.* New York: National League for Nursing.

Holloway, N. M.(1988). *Nursing the critically ill adult* (3rd ed.). Menlo Park, CA: Addison-Wesley.

Hudak, C. M., Gallo, B. M., and Lohr, T. (1986). *Critical care nursing: A holistic approach* (4th ed.). Philadelphia: Lippincott.

Kenner, C. V., Guzzetta, C.E., and Dossey, B. M. (1985). *Critical care nursing: Body-mind-spirit* (2nd ed.). Boston: Little, Brown.

Kinney, M. R., Packa, D. R., & Dunbar, S. B. (1986). *AACN's clinical reference for critical care nursing* (2nd ed.). New York: McGraw-Hill.

Reed S. B., & Hoffman, S. E. (1986). The enigma of graduate nursing education: Advanced generalist? Specialist? *Nursing & Health Care, 7*(1), 43-49.

U.S. Department of Health and Human Services. (1988). *Sixth report to the president and congress on the status of health personnel in the United States.* (Report No. HRS-P-OD-88-1). Washington, DC: U.S. Government Printing Office.

Response to AACN Position Statements: The Clinical Practice Perspective

Vernice Ferguson

Societal needs and consumer demands continue to escalate, exceeding any one discipline's response to them. Increasingly, the regulation of the health care delivery system by government and the active engagement of corporate purchasers of health care are cogent reminders that realism must prevail among nurses as nursing is practiced. To declare or even assume that nursing education programs through the revision of curriculum alone will "ensure that graduates are prepared to meet society's health care needs" is a presumptuous notion.

The practice setting is becoming increasingly complex, dynamic, and stressful for today's clinicians. The phenomenal growth of knowledge, the proliferation of new technologies, and the ability to sustain life for an extended number of years for many remind us of some of the awesome challenges awaiting the student and the new graduate - more often than not, the young among us. Amidst our machines, pharmaceutical, and subspecialty-trained physicians and other health care providers, we now bring an expectation that baccalaureate students should be required to grasp critical care content and engage in related clinical experiences in the baccalaureate nursing program. I question whether they are ready to assume the awesome expectations of critical care nursing, a specialty area. I also question that our decision to make such demands on them is professionally, ethically, and personally sound. A conference such as this enables us to debate these issues and, it is hoped, reach agreement on the critical ones.

We speak of the practice of nursing as an art and a science. We plead for humanistic nursing practice and count on nurses to care for the whole person — not a body part, an organ, or a system. We observe more often than we would like the environment in which critical care nurses function as a demanding and, quite often, a chaotic one. The intensity and rapid pace of this practice environment often mitigate against advancing the art as well as the science of nursing, which embodies holistic and humanistic care. It is neither in the student's best interest nor in the patient's to require one who is preparing at the baccalaureate level for generalist nursing practice to engage in a critical care program or study and clinical experience.

Pressures abound from students, faculty members, and alumni, and many other interested parties within and beyond academe to influence curriculum design. Competing demands and interests, whether financial, philosophical, discipline - or program-specific, for example continually are being reconciled as the debate is engaged on the skills and knowledge to be acquired in a baccalaureate program. Nursing as it prepares its students for the real world of practice is highly susceptible to responding to the prevailing need of that moment in its desire to be responsive to the public.

My plea is to plan a curriculum with outcomes focused on assisting the student to do the following:

- Reason critically.
- Communicate with clarity, orally and in writing.
- Make ethical and aesthetic judgements.
- Develop beginning understandings of the social, economic, political, and professional issues raised by scientific research, the development of technology and it transfer, and a rapidly aging population.
- Understand one's role as a citizen, not only of this nation but of the world.

A principal goal of baccalaureate education is to ensure a broadly educated person. The arts and sciences offer much to be learned in any rigorous baccalaureate program. Competing with the need for an educated person in today's baccalaureate program is the requirement that the nursing student acquire a level of mastery of subjects such as anatomy, physiology, pathology, and pharmacology. New fields continue to emerge that greatly influence the practice of clinicians in the health sciences. Bioethics and bioengineering are principal among them. In each of these fields, on the basis of discoveries and advances of the last decade alone, students in a baccalaureate program require a great deal of information to ensure a contemporary nursing practice.

Hard choices must be made. As someone in the practice setting, I would prefer the solid grounding of the student in understanding the healthy organism and deviations from it, including the influence of external factors such as the environment and life-style. The nurse that I expect to receive from the baccalaureate nursing program is one who has been prepared for beginning practice in an acute care hospital setting as a generalist. I do not consider critical care nursing generalist practice, rather specialty nursing practice. The requisite knowledge, skills, and attitudes required for practice in the critical care environment would be acquired at the postbaccalaureate level, building on the firm foundation acquired in a solid baccalaureate program. The critical care environment is a rich one for nurses to provide leadership in ethical decision making and research specific to the problems encountered. Much has been written in recent years about needless laboratory tests and other procedures. Can we look to critical care nurses, the constant and skilled monitors of care, to offer answers from their research? Can we also look to these nurses to extend the work of Knaus and his colleagues on the critical determinants of decreased morbidity and mortality in ICUs? (Knaus, 1986) What information can critical care nurses provide as they question existing protocols, policies, and procedures that have no basis in fact? Nurses prepared in this specialty area at the postbaccalaureate level can offer much.

The Faculty-Service Interface

All too often in the practice setting we have unrealistic expectations of the new graduate from the baccalaureate program in nursing. It is equally unrealistic in a practice discipline such as nursing to find faculty members whose credibility as practitioners in an area in which they teach is wanting. It is fortunate when faculty members seek and find practice settings in which the proficiency of the clinical nurses ensures an acceptable clinical experience for students. Many "practice experts," employees of the institution, assume responsibility for the student as they guide the student's clinical experience without being integral in any other way to the mission of the educational institution. It is lamentable, however, to note how often these competent clinicians, to whom educators entrust students, are denied faculty appointments in acknowledgment of their expert clinical knowledge and skills that they impart to students.

Some comparisons that highlight significant differences in medical education deserve our attention. Generally, the medical student is a product of a classic baccalaureate education. Medical school education provides didactic teaching from a broad array of disciplines, primarily the sciences, and limited clinical experience is offered under supervision. Residency training provides the resident physician with a well-supported group of role models, teachers, and mentors, some of whom are nurses. Specialty training and independent performance are not expected of the new medical school graduate, who more often is an older person and one with a longer educational experience than is the case with the new graduate in nursing. A more consistent and expected support system is in place for resident physicians as they practice and integrate what was learned in medical school in the practice environment as patients are cared for.

The Educated Nurse and the Knowledge Explosion

What should we strive for in educating the future nurse in a baccalaureate program? I suggest the following are of critical importance as we assist the student in becoming an "educated person," one who will practice in a clinical discipline:

- Development of problem-solving, observation, and assessment skills.
- Ability to relate to and teach consumers of nursing and health care services as they are prepared for discharge and independent or less dependent status.
- Beginning acumen in functioning as a direct care provider and team. member in an organized health care delivery system.

The basic body of knowledge in all disciplines continues to grow and at a phenomenal rate. Even experts find it difficult to keep abreast of advancements in their own field, much less in other fields. John Kemeny, President of Dartmouth, was asked, What is an educated person? A summary of his comments (Kemeny, Miller, Gregorian, 1980) and that of others appeared in the *New York Times*. When asked, What is now demanded when we call for an educated person? John Kemeny replied that the greatest need was still for breadth of education. He contended that this need was greater than it was 10 or 20 years earlier. In particular, he contended that "we desperately need individuals who can pull together knowledge from a wide variety of field and integrate it into one mind."

I have cited Dr. Kemeny for I share his view of what is expected of an educated person and extend his comments as I question our unrealistic expectations of the new graduate from a baccalaureate educational program. This graduate should be prepared as a generalist. This becomes even more germane as we confront a monumental shortage of nurses, primarily in hospitals. This shortage is expected to continue into the 21st century as the demand for nursing services continues. Some of the concerns that make nursing practice in hospitals less attractive for many nurses are related to the intensity of the environment, the multiple demands placed on the nurse, and inadequate support systems. With the diminished pool of young persons for whom we compete fiercely at issue, it is incumbent on us to ensure more care in taking care of new graduates as they prepare for careers in nursing. A baccalaureate curriculum that continues to respond unrealistically to the complex health care needs and requirements of a demanding public, along with a questioning society regarding the quality of a college education should cause us to pause. We must remind ourselves that we cannot be all things to all people for all times.

Integration and the Task Ahead

The Random House College Dictionary (1986) defines integrate as to "bring together or incorporate (parts) into a whole." An observation is in order as we reach back into our history in the educational preparation for professional nursing practice. At an earlier time in curriculum development, we spoke of integrating mental health and rehabilitation concepts throughout the curriculum. Some nurse leaders have suggested that we integrated mental health and rehabilitation nursing "out of the curriculum," leaving students without the conceptual knowledge or basic skills to practice with confidence. It appears that in our zeal to get everything in we succeeded in watering down specialty-specific information, making it utterly useless. Special care should be taken to avoid this occurrence in the baccalaureate curriculum as concepts related to critical care nursing are taught.

Rather than an attempt at refining the content or adding even more, a larger agenda is in order. That agenda becomes one of agreement in nursing on the expectations of the graduate of a baccalaureate program in nursing, the definition of generalist and specialty nursing practice, and models of parity for nurses in education and practice as we unify nursing, a clinical practice discipline.

Significant progress already has been made by the American Association of Colleges of Nursing in their final report, *Essentials of College and University Education for Professional Nursing*, funded by the Pew Memorial Trust in 1986. Twelve abilities to be acquired by a liberally educated professional nurse and seven values considered essential for the professional nurse leave little room it seems to me for specialty education at the baccalaureate level.

The need to reach agreement on the larger agenda, what should baccalaureate education encompass, requires our attention. Let us get on with the task.

References

American Association of Colleges of Nursing. (1986). *Essentials of college and university education for professional nursing final report*. Washington, D.C.: Author.

Kemeny, J., Miller, G., & Gregorian, V. (1980, May 18). What is an educated person? *New York Times*.

Knaus, W. A., Draper, E. A., Wagner, D. P., & Zimmerman, J. E. (1986). An evaluation of outcome from intensive care in major medical centers. *Annals of Internal Medicine, 104*, 410-418.

Random House College Dictionary. (3rd ed.). (1986). New York: Random House, (p. 692).

Response to Hawken and Ferguson: An Educator's Response

Sandra B. Dunbar

When the position statement advocating inclusion of critical care nursing in the baccalaureate curriculum was developed by AACN (1987), it seemed crystal clear to me that this needed to happen. The overwhelming increase in demand for critical care nursing services over the last decade mandates that we introduce our beginning practitioners to critical care nursing.

Vernice Ferguson has asked, "What is realistic?" One aspect of reality is that nurses with baccalaureate degrees are being employed in critical care. As an educator, I am concerned with the great variability in the preparation of critical care nurses. Although an impressive 95% of universities surveyed by AACN and NLN reported inclusion of critical care nursing in their curricula, the variability of the content and clinical experiences is disturbing. The majority of critical care nursing education is actually provided by hospitals.

The debate over generalist vs. specialist preparation at the baccalaureate level seems almost moot at this point when we examine the realities of nursing practice, in particular, the hospital setting. The spiraling level of activity in the inpatient setting has been discussed in detail and acknowledged at gatherings of nursing leaders across the United States. In conversations with hospital administrators, it becomes increasingly clear that any efforts to downsize hospitals do not include plans for decreasing the number of beds in critical care units. On the contrary, most institutions project growth in critical care areas. And, despite the American public's intrigue with fitness and prevention of illness, there is *no* evidence that the number of patients requiring critical care is declining. New programs in transplantation and neonatal care and sophisticated trauma and life-support networks all create more categories of patients who need the special knowledge and skills of critical care nurses.

How will the nursing profession meet the challenge of preparing critical care nurses? We have several options. We can continue in our current mode, that is, having no consistency and letting hospitals bear almost the *total* burden and expense of providing didactic and clinical preparation. Or, we can say critical care is technical care and should be performed by registered care technicians. I personally do not want to be at the other end of an endotracheal tube if that is our choice. Or, we can say that the baccalaureate curriculum is too full and bulging as is. We have a hard time designating anything to be removed from the curriculum. Thus, we can take a stand that all critical care nurses should be prepared at the Master's level — a position certainly not grounded in reality. None of these will do.

Let me pose another unpopular question. Will there be a place for a medical-surgical or adult health generalist in the near future? The increasing application of critical care nursing skills and knowledge outside the walls of the traditional critical care unit has blurred and will continue to blur the boundaries of acute and critical care nursing.

I wholeheartedly support the strategy of the Secretary's Commission on Nursing (1988) to reformulate our academic curricula to reflect the realities of the time. We must reexamine contemporary nursing practice and those components of nursing that can be generalized to more than one setting. I remember learning to palpate a fundus in an undergraduate obstetric course. I have not practiced in an obstetric setting since my basic education 17 years ago, but having cared for obstetric patients brought to the ICU in crisis. I am glad I was taught the why's, what's, and how's of this practice. I submit to you that our graduates who practice nursing in the general hospital today need to know basic concepts of electrocardiography and interpretation of dysrhythmias, hemodynamics and assessment, aspects of human interfacing with technology, caring for families in crises, and the ethical issues created by starting and terminating certain life-sustaining measures. These are a few examples of critical care nursing concepts that should be identified by the academic-service team and incorporated into nursing education. And, never has the need been greater for collaboration between academia and service.

In each of Vernice Ferguson's reasons *not* to include this so-called specialty content, I find underscored reasons to do so. As she explains so eloquently, an educated person is one with "breadth of experience who can pull together knowledge from different fields and integrate it into one mind." How can a nurse be educated today if a critical piece of knowledge is missing? Ms. Ferguson challenges our decision to integrate critical care nursing concepts and clinical experiences on the basis of personal, professional, and ethical soundness. I disagree and wonder how professionally and ethically sound it is to continue to graduate students who are unprepared for the realities they are to face in the hospital and even home care settings.

Incorporating critical care nursing will have another positive benefit for academic nursing programs, for I think it will increase the marketability of any particular nursing program and its graduates. As nursing programs compete for students in a declining pool of applicants, a program with critical care components may attract those who already have a designated interest in acute and critical care. In addition, these programs may attract the collaborative support of institutions willing to fund scholarships.

On a peripheral subject, I would like to respond also to a pervasive undercurrent found in many of the papers prepared for this conference. Many of our nursing leaders tend to equate critical care nursing with care of technology. These misconceptions about what nursing does with technology are disturbing. Ms. Ferguson even suggests that the critical care practice environment "often mitigates against advancing the art as well as the science of nursing, which embodies holistic and humanistic care."

I disagree — for it is the critical care nurse who serves as the *sole* caring, human link among the critically ill patients, their life-support technology, and their families. Physicians treat respiratory failure with oxygen, drugs, and mechanical ventilation. In addition to managing the technologic aspects, critical care nurses diagnose and treat the *human responses* of the patient, which might include positioning and hydration to mobilize secretions, protecting the airway, ensuring nutrition adequate to support respiratory muscle function, creating an alternative mode for communicating with the patient, providing explanations and hope for the family, and helping the family support the patient.

Consumers may settle for more affordable or reasonable choices when purchasing a car, but when it comes to health care that want — and demand — the best in technology and nursing. It is high time for nursing to embrace technology and health care and develop 20th and 21st century attitudes. The cost of not doing so is grave indeed, and it will result in lost opportunities. One of these is the opportunity to attract bright young scientists to the profession. The next generation of nurses is far ahead of us in computer literacy, and they place high values on technologic adjuncts in society and health. Continuing to denigrate nursing's role in the application of technology may cause us to lose potential students, or may result in the creation of more technicians. Another opportunity that might be lost is the opportunity to advance the health and welfare of humans. Nursing needs to raise pertinent questions about the appropriate application of technology. To do so, we must understand technology, participate in the decisions regarding its use, and be knowledgeable enough to raise the right questions. Nursing also must study human responses to health care technology as the technology is developed, not 10 to 15 years later, as we are doing now.

To summarize my points, first I think it is imperative that we provide an introduction to critical care nursing at the baccalaureate level by reexamining contemporary nursing practice and identifying those critical care concepts that have emerged and become more applicable outside the critical care unit.

Second, I challenge nursing faculty members and clinical practitioners involved in curriculum development to reexamine the content related to the care of patients across the patients' life span, and its relevancy, and to work together to create critical care learning opportunities for baccalaureate nursing students. By this challenge, I am not advocating that the outcome be an advanced critical care specialist, but rather a well-educated beginning generalist who has the ability to apply critical care nursing knowledge in an increasingly complex world of patient care.

Third, because technology is an integral part of our existing and future health care system, I challenge us to remember that *caring and technology* are symbiotic for our critically ill patients. Neither can exist without the other. I subscribe to the thought posed by Rene Dubos, who said, "We must not ask where science and technology are taking us, but rather how we can use science and technology to get where we want to go."

Finally, I wish to thank Patty Hawken for seeking clarification and posing some strategies and requesting more specific resources. It sounds as if AACN has a lot of work to do. I wish to thank Vernice Ferguson for her eloquent and, as always, provocative comments and for not acquiescing to the host position. It is only through clear articulation of the issues and open debate that our goal of consensus will be reached.

References
American Association of Critical-Care Nurses. (1987). *Need for critical care content and clinical experiences in baccalaureate nursing curricula* (AACN position statement) Newport Beach, CA: Author.

Secretary's Commission on Nursing. (1988). *Final report* (Vol. I). Washington, D.C.: Department of Health and Human Services.

Response to Hawken and Ferguson: A Clinical Manager's Response

Linda D. Searle

I would like to thank both presenters for their thoughts and analyses of AACN's position on integration of critical care content into the baccalaureate curriculum. There is much to be learned from both of them. It is clear that there are many areas of agreement.

One of the key elements in Dr. Hawken's presentation was the idea for the need to determine the essential content. This is an astute and important approach. We must be sensitive to the ever growing demands for an expanded curriculum. It is essential to prioritize what absolutely must be in a baccalaureate curriculum.

Dr. Hawken posed the question, "How does a specialty group influence faculty members to address content and clinical experiences within a specialty?" As the president of our association, I would like to take a moment and respond to this question. AACN monitors (and influences) the environment. AACN monitors the clinical areas in which we practice our specialty. Through this process, we identify issues, changes, and the technology that affects how we practice — aspects of the environment that affect our ability as critical care nurses to deliver care to critically ill patients. AACN comprehensively monitors the environment on an annual basis and conducts longer range planning for 3 to 5 years. In carrying out such an environmental analysis over the past few years, we have found that the preparation needs of critical care nurses remains an issue. We, as an association, continue to address many of these needs, but overall this remains an unresolved aspect of our specialty. There is a role for associations to play: a central role in identifying the needs within the practice setting.

An area I mentioned earlier is the increasing demand for more curriculum time. We must maintain our sensitivity to these increasing demands. There is, however, so much to be excited about in nursing. As we think about preparing nurses for practice, we want our own areas of interest captured in the curriculum. Some of these areas we indeed would want to teach and to ensure that others are learning about as well. However, the continuing demands for more curriculum time reflect the needs that exist in practice. Some of these needs are based on new knowledge being generated and some are the result of the information society that we have become. Our educational systems must be able to respond to changing practice needs such as these.

Our curricula must respond to the current and future context of hospital nursing. Data indicate that the majority of patients are more acutely ill than ever before. The occupancy rates in critical care continue to increase. Patients enter critical care units with more multiple systems failure than in the past. Patients' lengths of stay are shorter; they transfer to medical and surgical areas sooner. The hospital setting has become more intense, and the increased demand for critical care nurses is projected to continue (AACN, 1988). The design of baccalaureate nursing curricula must address these changes.

Most importantly, I offer a response on the definition of critical care. Dr. Hawken asked, "Is it a place? Is it an environment? Is it a role?" Yes, it is all of those things. AACN has defined critical care nursing through a position statement title on *AACN Scope of Critical Care Nursing Practice* (AACN, 1986). This statement depicts a conceptual model and reflects the interactive nature of three elements: the patient, the nurse, and the environment. All three must exist for critical care nursing to exist. Confusion may result when we look at a definition such as the one from the Department of Health and Human Services. It is an accurate definition of critical care but what is missing for me in that definition of critical care is the nursing component. AACN's statement on the scope of practice contains the definition of critical care nursing that is built on the ANA's definition of nursing. We cannot separate our specialty from professional nursing practice. However, what needs to be emphasized most at this point is the critically ill patient's primary need for physiological stability. A patient who is physiologically unstable enters the critical care environment because a potentially life-threatening need exists. There are many patients, such as a severely obese patient or a patient threatening suicide, who's current health state does not involve physiological instability of a life-threatening nature. Certainly these are serious situations, but they do not require admission to a critical care unit. A second point is that patients with physiological instability require a critical care nurse. The critical care nurse provides comprehensive assessment and intervention.

The AACN Certification Corporation completed a role delineation study (Sullivan, Sanford, & Samph, 1988) that was used as the blueprint for certification examination. It is really a job analysis of the role of the critical care nurse. This is an additional reference that further adds to the definition of critical care nursing. AACN's *Core Curriculum* (Alspach & Williams, 1985) contains the body of knowledge identified as essential in order to practice at a competent level and demonstrate specialized knowledge of critical care nursing. The role of the critical care nurse is further defined by AACN *Standards for Nursing Care for the Critically Ill* (Sanford & Disch, 1989).

I also would like to address some of my comments to the issues that Ms. Ferguson has raised. I mentioned that the number of critical care beds is increasing. Occupancy rates in critical care are rising. The length of the patient's stay is shorter. We would be denying reality if we did not recognize that hospital nursing is changing and that we must begin to prepare nurses for that changing environment. Yes, it is a demanding environment and perhaps hospital nursing itself is a unrealistic event for a new graduate, a new nurse. Yet, it is reality. Therefore, I think it demands our support, our increased attention, and our "intensive care" to provide support for entering nurses that facilitates their role development, smooth their transition, and helps them be as successful as they can be, as successful as we need them to be.

Many of our current practitioners have come from associate degree programs. This is another reality that we must recognize. Nurses who are delivering critical care nursing today have not learned their specialty from postbaccalaureate education. We need to address this reality, not leave it unattended. Critical care courses are provided in the hospital setting, and yet hospitals are cutting their resources more than ever before. I am not sure that we can expect 6-to-8 week critical care preparatory entrance courses to continue. Are we content with that possibility?

And last, I am concerned that we might think it is not in the best interest of the patient to prepare the critical care nurse by means of the baccalaureate curriculum. First and foremost, what is not in the best interest of our patients is not having an adequate number of prepared critical care nurses to care for critically ill patients and the patients' families.

References

Alspach, J. G. & Williams, S. M. (1985). *Core Curriculum for Critical Care Nursing* (3rd ed.). Philadelphia: W. B. Saunders.

American Association of Critical-Care Nurses. (1986). *AACN Scope of Practice*. Newport Beach, CA.

American Association of Critical-Care Nurses. (1988). *Summary analysis of critical care nurses supply and requirements*. Newport Beach, CA: Author.

Sanford, S., & Disch, J. M. (1989). *Standards for nursing care of the critically ill* (2nd ed.). San Mateo, CA: Appleton & Lange.

Sullivan, S., Sanford, S., & Samph, T. (1988). *Final report: Content and construction validation of the CCRN certification examination 1982-1984*. Newport Beach, CA: AACN Certification Corporation.

SECTION 2
Realities and Trends in Baccalaureate Education

Performance Expectations of New Graduates

Patricia Benner

Preparing this paper was more of a challenge than I had expected. First, it seems patently obvious to me that we need major resource allocations, to prepare nurses to practice in critical care units at the undergraduate, graduate, and professional continuing education levels, and that a sound basis for this progression must begin at the baccalaureate level. So why would anyone be asked to write a position statement on the obvious? Answering this question led me to consider what an enormous accomplishment critical care nurses and their educators have made in a short time with limited, almost nonexistent space, money, and time. In a mere 30 years, nurses have developed a highly specialized practice that is unique in health care, and they have done this with little visibility, few resources and little recognition. This feat often has been accomplished with little respect for the impact these difficult lessons have had on the learner. Others have assumed that we could do it with few resources, little time, and minimal teaching, and we have met this challenge but with great collective and personal cost. I think that the broader purpose of this conference is to point to our accomplishment and to set about to get the money, resources, and time to do the job with less personal cost to the learner and to the practicing teachers both in academia and in the clinical setting. To do this, I will examine why and how of critical care nursing is so invisible that we sources for education needed to prepare baccalaureate nurses for this practice.

Causes of Invisibility

Intensive care nursing practice has a peculiar cultural covering over and invisibility. In a current study, sponsored by the Helene Fuld Foundation, on the development of clinical knowledge and expert clinical judgment of intensive care unit nurses, we are examining the sources of the invisibility and marginality of this central life-saving practice.* Ultimately, making the expert knowledge and practice of critical care nursing visible and understood is a historical task, a research and development task, a clinical knowledge development task, and finally a curricular task.

As a field of study, expert knowledge in intensive care nursing is relatively new, roughly 30 years old. It has developed largely in an ad hoc, delegated, practice-based fashion. To clarify the base of this knowledge development, we can contrast intensive care nursing practice with the space program, which largely has been a theoretical enterprise with a great deal of planning: underwritten costs; public, governmental, and private attention; and lavish attention on the practitioners of space, the astronauts. Intensive care practice and the cornerstone of that practice, nursing, have been accomplished by an invisible women's profession, with almost no recognition; almost no formal funding; little large-scale systematic planning; and finally with a now familiar illegitimate authority, indirect power, and pattern of status inequity.

Hospitals have become increasingly focused on intensive care. Therapies are instantaneous, most often involve intravenous administration, and require astute instantaneous clinical judgment. The style of physicians orders has switched from precise mandates to guidelines that instruct the nurse to keep the patient within certain physiological limits and within certain therapeutic dosage ranges of medication based on the patient's responses. This change in nursing practice began in the intensive care units, but now is common in every hospital unit. Indeed, the judgment about whether a patient needs to be in the hospital is based on whether the patient needs instantaneous treatments carefully watched and managed by nurses

---

* This study is sponsored by a grant from the Helene Fuld Foundation. Catherine Chesia, RN, DNSc and Susan Thollaug, RN, MS, are acknowledged for their assistance in the background analysis for this paper.

or whether the treatment can be administered safely, with less clinical judgment, in the home.

The invisibility in this extraordinary practice seems to have many causes. I focus here on nine that have become evident in our preliminary analysis. These sources will be refined further and examined critically in our study of the practice of intensive care nurses at the beginning, competent, and expert levels.

Giving Legitimacy to Knowledge that is Formal, Abstract, and General, while Devaluing and Overlooking Knowledge that Is Local, Specific, and Based in Practice and Skill

Dreyfus and Dreyfus (1986; also, Dreyfus, 1979) point out that the Western tradition has a systematic error that began with Plato and Socrates. Knowledge, if it was to count as knowledge in this early Greek account, had to be capable of being decontextualized, generalized, and abstracted to cover a range of situations. This theoretical formal property became privileged in the Western tradition so that knowledge came to mean abstract, general, principled, systematic information that can be applied to a wide range of situations. In this view, knowledge is generated and then applied to chaotic situations. This view lent itself easily to Descartes's further tenet that knowledge is privatized in a subject's mind and applied to an objectified world (Benner & Wrubel, 1989; Dreyfus, in press; Heidegger, 1982). The legacy of this view can be seen easily in critical care nursing practice. The physician's orders are written in terms of parameters or limits, and these broad principles are considered knowledge with a capital K, whereas the mere working out of that knowledge with specific patients is just a procedural carrying out of the principle. It does not take long to figure out that an enormous knowledge gap exists between the principle and the practice. For example, critical care nurses talk eloquently about fields of tension between over- and undermedicating. Questions and judgments are rampant: Is this a transitory rise in blood pressure due to movement, or does it signal the beginning of a trend that requires additional medication? In a postoperative open heart patient, is the increased heart rate due to early signs of cardiac decompensation, high blood sugar, or low fluid volume? Critical care nurses talk about qualitative distinctions providing the encouragement and structure to help patients cope with intrusive and painful procedures and the violation of a patient's rights to refuse those treatments: Is this patient shutting down and shutting everyone out as a way of coping with despair, pain, and exhaustion, or is this an early sign of septic shock?

I will not proliferate the thousands of judgment questions that are the minute-by-minute content of critical care nursing practice. My point is that we must acknowledge that it is a dangerous cultural blindness to assume that the abstract knowledge is knowledge with a capital K and that practice-based clinical knowledge of the particular is lesser knowledge. This error causes us to overlook the skilled knowledge and judgment required in the practice, and causes us to prepare nurses inadequately to make these judgments.

Furthermore, we do violence to our expert knowledge when we think of the patient and the clinical situation as chaotic, having no order, meaning, and coherence on its own. The expert clinician always is trying to understand what dysrhythmias and cardiac outputs any particular patient can tolerate as a result of the patient's adaptation over time. This knowledge of the particular is not chaotic noninformation: It is the essential base for all critical care nursing judgments. We do violence to patients when we do not take seriously the order and the bodily adaptive capacities that they bring to us. We have to find ways to bring this kind of clinical knowledge to the forefront of both medicine and nursing.

Separating Means from Ends and Devaluing the "Mere" Means

The separation of means from ends is being discovered as a major pedagogical problem in mathematics, science, and technology (Benner, 1984 Collins, 1985; Dreyfus & Dreyfus, 1986; Lave, 1988).

Algorithmic problem solving is assumed to be the ideal model for the cognitive procedures employed to solve questions of fact in the service of goals exogenous to the process under study. This view isolates action as technique, and knowledge as "fact" from ends as matters of value, desire, feeling, and judgment. Indeed, the concept of "goals" is merely the obverse of "problem solving procedures." Both result from the single stroke that divides means from ends, fact from value.(p.174)

The separation of means and ends assumes that the practice of critical care nursing is a mere technology, that is, a mere application of abstract, formal knowledge that can be applied, as if following the directions on a label. The separation of means and ends is a fallout of the view of knowledge as abstract and formal, but it deserves special attention because it is such a pervasive and insidious source of the invisibility in critical care nursing practice. Albert Borgmann (1984) has pointed out that a technological approach to knowledge is not just a problem of separating means and ends, but that we do violence to our practices when means and ends are not considered together. All means are not equal. Some means may accomplish an outcome but do violence to the ends in the process.

The separation of means and ends lends itself to the problem of means ends displacement, that is, means become more important, and efficiency unwittingly becomes the end, displacing more important ends. This was brought home to me in a powerful way when I was a visiting scholar at Beth Israel Hospital in Boston. I participated in rounds in the coronary care unit where the last patient was discussed in hushed reverent tones. She was "doing her best to die" but was lingering, in a semiconscious state. The family was at her side, and no more heroic measures were reasonable. I was struck by the involvement, of staff members, both physicians and nurses, and by the compassionate care I saw. I could not help but ask, thinking I had fallen into a time warp, why this woman was still in the ICU inasmuch she was dying. The nurses and physicians alike looked at me and my question with horror and incredulity and answered, "We do not think that it would be fair to the family or to the staff to move her at this point. We just could not do it. It would be a kind of abandonment." I responded, "I agree, but how do you manage? Do you always do this? What if you needed her bed for a critically ill patient?" They responded in a wonderfully humane, nonrational way (notice I said nonrational, not irrational), "Well, it's a little like family. Once the commitment is there, there always seems to be room." In this era of commercialization and bottom-line health care, they had managed not to confuse outcome with worthy ends. They still have a lively discussion about worthy ends, but that has not deteriorated into a separation of means from ends or a discourse on efficiency . They are clear that they do violence to themselves and their patients when they abandon the dying patient through efficient bureaucratic transfer.

I think that if we understand the knowledge embedded in expert critical care nursing practice, we will have to develop new management strategies. Here I want to quote from Benner & Wrubel (1989).

Managerial language and practices that seek to objectify, quantify and decontextualize conflict with the nature of caring practices. Patients feel cared for when they are not treated as merely "customers," "consumers" or "resources." When we are ill, we want to feel cared for. Even the most autonomous modern wants to confidently trust that humane, sensitive care will be available if he were incapacitated, unable to be assertive or demand rights. The notion of the self in opposition to others and an ethic limited to rights and justice cannot account for caring for another who cannot exert full powers except in "paternalistic" terms. An ethic of relatedness, care and responsibility is needed to account for the mutual trust required for caring for the incapacitated. Caring practices in the context of familial and community membership need not be paternalistic. A culture that emphasizes independence and individualism cannot survive without a safety net of care and caring practices. The rational-technical model of management has no language or strategies for determining what are worthy goals (MacIntyre, 1981; March, 1976). The rational-technical model is limited to the assumption that we know what are the appropriate ends and that the only problem is how to be more efficient in reaching pre-determined ends. To go beyond the rational-technical model we need to develop a discourse on worthy ends. (p. 399)

We are finding a rich discourse on worthy ends embedded in expert critical care nursing, and this is one of the promising lines of interpretation in the current study of expert knowledge in critical care. This ethic of expert critical care nursing practice departs from traditional biomedical ethics, which tend to be problem centered (focused on iatrogenic problems that raise new questions of autonomy and rights). This analysis awaits further collection of data but the critical care nurses talk about how patients ought to be cared for, the failures and dilemmas of care, and the patient's network of care. This discourse has the potential for forming a basis for a substantive ethic of care and responsibility for the acutely ill and disadvantaged.

Assuming that Knowledge Is Atomistic, Elemental, and Procedural and thus Overlooking Relational, Configurational, and Embodied Knowledge

Expert critical care knowledge contains many discrete elements of knowledge, but these discrete elements, the numbers, never tell the whole story; indeed, in isolation, they tell very little. And yet the lore of the rational-technical model is that numbers are the story. I think that schools need to spearhead an effort to increase the teaching capacities of schools of nursing to prepare nurses to understand thoroughly the major commonly used technology in critical care. However, from the beginning, that knowledge must be related to the particular patient and to the relational and configurational context for interpreting the numbers. Clearly this requires a strong emphasis on pathophysiology, hemodynamic monitoring, and the pathophysiological alterations common with unconsciousness and with compromised cardiovascular systems. However, even this formal knowledge, though necessary, will not be sufficient. Clinical instruction that associates formal indicators with actual signs and symptoms is needed also. Clinical learners spend a great deal of time relating external signs and symptoms to formal indicators, and this process could be made more systematic and focused. For example, in our study of expert clinical judgment in critical care, a nurse described learning to recognize and relate the physical appearance and signs and symptoms of respiratory distress in an infant with the formal physiological measurements of pH and CO_2:

> NURSE: *The child was in a horrible respiratory state, and they did not want to intubate him because of the possible repercussions. His lungs were so fragile at that point that they could blow a pneumo or cause more problems and scarring. He had been intubated once before, so they were trying to keep him from being intubated. The child had a primary diagnosis of hypoplastic lung and bilateral hydronephrosis. [As it turned out, this child probably should have been intubated earlier, and might have been if an expert nurse had been caring for him. Other nurses wanted him intubated, but the action was blocked by disagreement among physicians. The child was intubated first thing in the morning. Here the point is to illustrate the necessary learning involved in associating physical signs of respiratory distress with physical measurements.] I was checking his blood gases constantly. He was in permanent metabolic acidosis, so you could see him compensating respiratorially throughout the night, and we were watching for any minor changes in that. When he was mildly sedated, he was more relaxed. His arm movements stopped, but he never was really good. The nasal flaring never stopped, the lips were smacking, and he was real focused. The signs that I wouldn't necessarily know, but as people came in, they would say: "See that, see the way he's moving his lips, see how he's kind of looking straight up into the ceiling as opposed to kind of looking around the room. These are all signs that this child is very focused and is taking everything he has to breathe." So watching signs like that, and when I saw that he relaxed his lips and when his hands stopped, when the retractions weren't quite as severe, that was when I knew he was not working quite as hard. His heart rate also came down, that sort of thing.*
>
> INTERVIEWER: *You said that you learned a lot that night, and you gave us some examples of how nurses and doctors pointed out things to observe. Is that a good way for you to learn?*
>
> NURSE: *Yes. I like to be able to see. And I know gases are important but you can't look at a child and know what his pH is. At least I can't. I'm sure*

> *maybe some people can. But for me, I can't, so I like to be able to recognize the external, the very obvious. That in time will come without me even thinking about it, but right now, I need all those little things pointed out to me. I think that's very helpful. I had never really seen a child using his body to breathe. And, he was really moving his arms in rhythm with his breaths. Really working at it. And the reason I hadn't seen it is because most of the kids are intubated and there is no effort involved there. There's more effort to fight the ventilator. It's so unusual for a child on the unit to be extubated.*

Note that the formal pathophysiological knowledge of respiratory distress is not sufficient for making a clinical judgment about the signs and symptoms of respiratory distress. The clinician must have a firm first-person grasp of what respiratory distress looks like in the infant. This is just the kind of learning that would yield to videotape instruction and focused observation on the unit for assessment of informal signs and symptoms in relation to formal physical measurements. Note, that if the graduate had had training in making the qualitative distinctions about respiratory distress in infants, he or she still would need to master the specific social system in order to get an appropriate response from the physician to a more refined ability to determine when someone needs respiratory assistance.

Learning the Relationships between Formal Procedural Knowledge and Practical Embodied Skill

Although it is essential to formalize, (i.e., make explicit and describe in procedural ways) all the critical care knowledge that can be made explicit and formalized, it is simply not possible to make explicit all the knowledge and judgment that are called forth in an open, indeterminate clinical situation. There are limits to procedural descriptions just as there are limits to knowledge that can be conveyed in formal doctor's orders (a misnomer that more appropriately should be called medical limits and guidelines). Here I want to use the description of skilled handling of fragile premature infants in whom oxygen desaturation often occur if they are handled at all. I quote a neonatal ICU nurse's expert description of handling premature infants and then her naive statement to me that she has written this embodied skill up in a descriptive procedure that other nurses can read and use. Now, although while the procedural description is essential for pointing out the knowledge, for making it visible, it is not sufficient for teaching the embodied skill of handling the infant, and it is a cultural blindness about the power of procedural descriptions and formalism that makes the nurse believe that such transfer is plausible. Of course, the nurse easily reads in her skill when she reads the procedural description; the uninitiated are left to their impoverished imagination:

> **FIRST NURSE:** *Also, I think that there's something to the fact that babies know when they are being handled by somebody who knows what he or she is doing and when they are not. I think babies get scared just like anyone else when someone is clearly nervous and clearly not as quick about hooking them back up to the ventilator, or clearly having a hard time getting a tube down.*
>
> **SECOND NURSE:** *Preemies never like to be handled. They almost never do. They just desaturate, and they cannot handle any kind of stimulation. So, I start out first of all by getting into the isolette quietly. I don't bang the portholes and make the baby jump a mile. I put a hand on the babies' back and just let them get used to the idea that I'm there and that I'm not hurting them. I always try to touch them, put my hands on and leave them there. I let them kind of squirm and figure out what they want to do with themselves. I usually stick their fingers in their mouths first thing, so that if they decide that they want to cry and be upset, they will have something in there to suck on. And usually they do.*
>
> **INTERVIEWER:** *You're prepared when you go in, and you have everything lined up that you need on hand?*
>
> **FIRST NURSE:** *You try to do everything and get out, close the door and do your charting. You don't just turn them over, you bring their knees into their chest and hold their arms at their sides so that they don't turn their back on you. It's reflexive that when you startle them, they are going to do that. It makes them very nervous. So you get them contained when you go to turn them. In fact, a lot of times when I first go to do vital signs, the first thing I will do is put the kid's feet inside the diaper to get small enough. You just Pamper (put the diaper on) them entirely up to their waists and get their legs inside, then you don't have to worry about them anymore. They can't kick around, and it makes them much happier. A lot of times I'll wrap a diaper around them or a blanket for the entire vital signs as much as I can, so that they don't flail around and so that they feel secure. It's just making them feel secure. That's all it is. It's so easy (laughter).*

(There is a discussion about how difficult it is to teach people how to do this.)

FIRST NURSE: *We have a small baby protocol with things like "Keep them in a flex position, keep blanket rolls around them so that they are in the nest and not sort of lying there flat on the back." We have instructions on shading the isolettes.*

There is much judgment, deftness, and recognition of similarities and differences in expert handling of preemies. And when these experts read the "protocol," they see things and read in their skills in ways that are simply impossible for the inexperienced beginner, or the competent nurse who has not yet learned the relationships between handling practices and the babies' physical responses.

Assuming that Knowledge Is Highly Compartmentalized and Specialized

In one view, expertise is equated with highly specialized, esoteric, compartmentalized knowledge. Nurses are the most numerous and most general health care practitioners in a highly specialized and diversified health care system. Let me quickly define what I mean by the "general" orientation of nursing. For example, the critical care nurse specialist is the most general of all the health care practitioners in critical care. Critical care nurses have highly specialized practices to attend to the relationships between health and sense of well-being, illness and disease in the acutely ill patient and the patient's significant others. Critical care nurses also see that the subspecialties in medicine and other therapists coordinate, communicate, and orchestrate their intent so that conflicting therapies, practices, or timing do not jeopardize the patient's well being. Nurses do this best because they understand the embodied patient and the relationships between physical states, conflicts between various therapeutic intents, social relationships, sense of well-being, and recovery. The highly specialized practice of critical care nursing is general in its approach even though the clinical judgment capacities of nurses are highly refined and specialized, and indeed are even the privileged domain of nurses (e.g., titrating pain medications and Pavulon, vasopressors, antidysrhythmic medications; weaning patients from respirators; understanding in a relational and configurational sense a particular patient's hemodynamics).

In the context of this highly specialized practice, critical care nursing is organized by the nurses' concern for and about their patients' and the patients' families' lived experience of illness. Even the most technical specialized practice in nursing is taken up on a background of concern about the lived experience of illness. Thus, in their highly specialized general approach, critical care nurse specialists bring something vital to the practice of high-tech health care. Critical care nurse specialists cannot be reduced to the level of mere technicians even though they must be exquisite technicians. It is the background caring practices that make nursing's contribution to high-tech critical care so essential for patients and families, and for society. This is demonstrated easily by many statements from ICU nurses in our current study of expert practice in ICUs. I quote a few to illustrate the point. For example, a new graduate discovers that the emphasis on psychosocial care was not a wasted school project after all.

> **FIRST NURSE:** *And it just struck me that I was taking care of this kid, and sometimes the family and parents need the nurses more than the patient does. . . I put on my kid gloves and tried to be as gentle as I could. I just tried to have a very reassuring tone because actually he [the baby] has a 90% chance, as far as these cases go. And I thought that was pretty good. . . I don't think nurses are as intimidating as physicians. No matter how nice a person you are, if you're a doc, just the role you take can sometimes be intimidating. And nurses just are more accessible to people I think. I don't know, maybe I'm biased.*
>
> **SECOND NURSE:** *No, I think part of that is, just nurses spend more actual time with the patient, they also spend more time with other physicians and aren't, maybe, as able to tone down their verbiage more and . . . just the way they present things. So, as we're used to speaking more with the parents, we are able to see what the parents can understand and what level of communication we can use to actually get the point across.*
>
> **FIRST NURSE:** *I think our level of training is so different too. In medical school, it's very — technical, and I've never been to medical school, so I can't say — but I think in nursing there's a little bit more emphasis and focus on holistic medicine. And when you're in nursing school, you're thinking, Yeah, right, lets just get to the meat and potatoes of this stuff. But when you get out into practice, it's true that you take a holistic approach to giving medical care or psychiatric care. (The nurse goes on to describe critical intervention with the family who really had not understood their baby's medical situation even though the baby was 3 weeks into a serious illness and 6 days postoperatively)*

With the general approach, and the diversity of the health care system, it is not surprising that nursing education faces pressure to be all things to all people. Indeed, one of the strengths of nursing is the diverse possibilities a nursing degree offers its holder. With great foresight, nursing educators long have discussed the problems of preparing the nurse for today and the future. Some might think that (1) care of illness and (2) wellness or health promotion are incompatible, but nursing ingeniously has understood that they are related. Nurses have understood that health cannot be reduced to a commodity, nor even to an all or none dichotomous variable.

This tradition of viewing health as containing a sense of well-being has persisted from the Nightingale period, when care was understood to be putting the patient's body in the best state to recover, to current nurse thinkers who view health as a continuum (Benner, 1984; Benner & Wrubel, 1989; Lynaugh & Fagin, 1988; Tripp-Reimer, 1984.) Nursing practice cannot be understood without understanding the wellness orientation that nursing holds. Nurses care about people's health, well-being, illness, disease, and recovery at whatever the point of contact is. Here I am making the common distinction between illness and disease, with illness being the human experience of loss or dysfunction associated with disease and disease being the pathophysiological breakdown at the organ, tissue, and cellular levels (Kleinman, Eisenberg & Good, 1978). Likewise, health is being defined as that which can be assessed physically and mentally, whereas well-being is the person's lived experience of health or wholeness (Benner & Wrubel, 1989).

Nurses are concerned about the relationship between health and well-being, between disease and illness. Nurses traditionally have had a strong commitment to rehabilitation, recovery, community health care, and health promotion in its broadest sense, and internationally, nurses have been charged with taking up the primary health care role. This concern for primary care, wellness, and health promotion is a second way in which nursing historically has had a general focus, though I think that this particular definition of general no longer works because the technical skills required in primary care and community care illustrate that we no longer can equate low technology with being general. A general approach, as I am defining it, means that the whole person in the context of family and community is considered in the caring practice, whether the person be well, ill, unborn, or dying, and that the relationships between illness and disease are considered. To understand health as a continuum, we must study the full range of the continuum. I think that we will not serve our role in primary health care, health promotion, and even in shaping and reshaping health care policy if we abandon our expert knowledge at the acute care end of the continuum of health care.

Ignoring the Human Side of Critical Care, Caring, Healing and Recovery

The focus of our current health care system has shifted from care to cure, despite the fact that many diseases are chronic and require care over time. The dominant view of the body in American medicine is mechanistic and focuses on cure. This is portrayed dramatically in ICUs, where the human side of illness, the desires and hopes for healing and recovery, may be exaggerated even more in the context of intrusive procedures, unnatural surroundings, and sleep deprivation. However, cure never is achieved without care, and cure requires healing and recovery. This tension over the invisibility and devaluation of the human side of care is evident in the previous quotation about the care needs of the family. For example, an ICU nurse said the following about weaning an extremely debilitated person who had suffered a stroke:

> But it was over a period of days making him comfortable with his weaning [from the respirator], and of making him psychologically comfortable, that he began showing improvement. Then his personality started to come out, and he was now willing to fight for his rehabilitation, willing to participate in his care. Really, our main thing is to psychologically keep him boosted enough so he can go through the weaning process.

A quotation from another nurse illustrates the common practice of giving the patients a say and empowering them in their caring practices. The patient's everyday activities become meaningful signals of hope, and of self-control:

> I always let them have even the smallest decisions — everything: "How do you like to be positioned? Would you rather me not do this?" Don't take things away from them. Sometimes it's faster for you to do things for them, but if you have the time, let them do that. It makes them feel like a human being. They think, "If I can still brush my own teeth, I must not be dying," or "It couldn't be that bad." Sometimes when we get the chronic patients, the problem is the other way around: It's making them take back control because they get so passive and so withdrawn. It's like forcing them to open their eyes and look at you, and nod to answer a question.

For these nurses, the technology of their work is relativized by the centrality of their caring practices, even though they are experts in making instantaneous adjustments of various intravenous medications and in warding off complications, and even though the technical aspects of their work take up much of their time.

Segregating the Work of Medicine and Nursing on the Basis of Sex

Much of the invisibility of nursing knowledge can be attributed to the fact that nursing is primarily a woman's profession. This, of course, is not a simple problem of translating women's knowledge, actions, and practices into male forms because the very forms are laden with content and knowledge. The discourse of diagnosis and cure is a language of mastery and control, and this discourse is often at odds with the intent and content of nurturing and care. Critical care nurses must come to terms with the dichotomies and with the tensions between cure and care in their practice. These tensions are made more difficult because curative intents may at times receive inappropriate value and attention, and the nurse may be doubly handicapped by status inequity in advocating curing or caring intents for the patient. Intensive care nurses make continual assessments and judgments about therapies, but this judgment is covered over by calling the medical guidelines orders as if they were clear directives to be carried out. The independent practice and unique skills are not fully sanctioned and legitimized. Much ambiguity exists. Therefore, when things go well, credit may be overlooked, and when things go wrong, the nurse may or may not be held accountable.

Assuming that Knowledge Is Only Private and Cognitive while Overlooking the Way Knowledge Is Embodied and Socially Embedded

Anthropologists and philosophers have been calling to our attention the ways knowledge is embodied and embedded in social practices (Benner, 1984; Benner & Tanner, 1987; Bourdieu, 1977; Collins, 1985; Dreyfus, 1979; Dreyfus & Dreyfus, 1986; Lave, 1988; Lock & Gordon, 1988; Merleau-Ponty, 1962; Polanyi, 1958; Suchman, 1987). This work has come from studying everyday practices in context. When complex skills are studied in the context of everyday practice, researchers and thinkers discover that groups as diverse as crystal growers, computer programmers, mathematicians, chess players, and nurses know more than the groups can tell and that the knowing and telling is contingent on the referential context of practice and complex embodied skills. It is essential to have the procedures and protocols described, but these do not capture adequately the decision points and the embodied know-how to make them work. This is a hard lesson for academia to learn. It is simply not possible to teach embodied and socially embedded skilled knowledge without clinical experience. And that clinical experience needs to be designed in safe and humane ways, so that neither the patient nor the learner suffers in the process. Bourdieu (1977) has pointed out that we will solve the problems inherent in the cultural blindness of thinking that the only choice lies between objectivism and subjectivism when we study the way people develop practical mastery in intelligible ways, while remaining enchanted by the indeterminate puzzles in open practical situations.

Hiding Demand Characteristics, and Responsibility as a Means of Defending against Anxieties Created by Life-and-Death Responsibilities

Menzies (1960) wrote an incredibly perceptive psychosocial analysis of the hospital that I think is equally relevant to critical care nursing practices. She pointed out that much of the bureaucratic dispersal and spreading of power and accountability in hospitals is an institutionally based defense against anxiety. Spreading the responsibility, that is, care through delegation and blurred boundaries between medical and nursing practices, covers over any one person's responsibility for the outcomes of life and death that occur hourly and daily in the ICU. I suspect that, in part, nurses have not clamored for more visibility of their awesome responsibility because they feel the responsibility heavily and would like to share it with others to ease the burden. This creates the temptation to take the credit for the successes, and to hide the failures. This use of invisibility as a defense against anxiety is an irrational and a dangerous practice. It does not protect a person effectively from the weight of responsibility and almost always buffers the credit and acknowledgment for success.

Many hours of observation and interviewing of critical care nurses over the past 15 years has convinced me that when a breakdown occurs, when a death or untoward response by the patient occurs that feels preventible, all sense of protection from responsibility accorded by delegation breaks down. Despite transitory assignments of blame, everyone feels equally responsible. Though the public disclaimers at the time may sound otherwise, I suspect that the private recriminations and reviews reveal a great sense of personal responsibility on the part of nurses and physicians. And I think that it cannot be otherwise for safe professional practice. I am convinced of this because of the many accounts of breakdown that have been reported to me in research interviews. These regrettable incidents may have occurred recently or as long as 5 and 10 years before, but they have been told to me as if they happened yesterday, and told in a way that indicates that the reporter is still working on ways to ensure that this *is* prevented next time. Personal responsibility is the core of professional accountability and the development of expert practice. We must guard against ineffective institutional and personal defenses against anxiety over this responsibility if our expert practice is to grow.

The Link between Invisibility and Lack of Legitimacy

When an expert practice lacks appropriate levels of visibility and legitimacy, it is hard to garner the educational resources needed (time, money, and expertise). Indeed, educational structures and processes are major legitimizing forces. A vicious circle develops: Lack of legitimacy breeds lack of educational space and resources and in turn creates further invisibility and lack of legitimacy. It is assumed that this "lesser knowledge," the mere carrying out of physicians' orders, easily can be taught on an ad hoc informal basis, requiring little formal time and space given to the education. Nowhere has this fallacy been more evident than in the infamous Registered Care Technician Proposal. This arrogant proposal assumes that anyone who has a little technical training can practice in critical care. The broad educational and moral base of the practice is overlooked, and a part task technology is the proffered replacement. For those whose practice is undervalued and relatively invisible, the possibility of hiding is ubiquitous, and hiding becomes a major tempting way of coping with the stresses, strains, and incredible responsibility of intensive care nursing practice.

Summary

The first step in coming to terms with what is possible to teach the undergraduate is to uncover the complexity and richness of the practice that we want to teach. I think that we can graduate advanced beginners who are well prepared to be astute clinical learners. I do not think it is possible to graduate "finished products" who can master the complexities of all the knowledge and judgment that is embedded in that practice. Technical mastery of the equipment and technology should be the easiest aspect to teach, and certainly it is important. However, we also must equip the new graduate to cope with the ethical dilemmas spawned by intensive care and highly technical medicine. We also must teach them to cope with caregiving and with bearing witness to great suffering. If we do not do a good job of teaching the human side, and the caring practice side, then our graduates will not be in a good position to be safe and human clinical learners and practitioners. We dare not hold up a model of technical proficiency without equal proficiency and understanding of our caring practices. We also dare not emphasize the general to the exclusion of the particular. Martha McDermott, neonatal intensive care nurse at The Children's Hospital, Boston, captured the role of the particular in clinical expertise well in describing her clinical expertise in neonatal intensive care:

"It is through our repeated experiences with patients that we begin to perceive the *particular* rather than the typical, care becomes *individualized* rather than standardized, and planning becomes *anticipatory* of change rather than simply responsive to change" (Benner & Wrubel, 1989, p. 382).

This describes the deep knowledge of the particular patient and the particular situation that the expert uses to orchestrate nursing care. The roles of the particular and "knowing how" vs. "knowing that" have a cultural stigma and blindness that have led us to not consider them knowledge at all. And that is a bias that we have to confront in academia. Our task now is to seek the resources, the time, the place, and the space to teach systematically this incredible body of knowledge that we have developed on a shoe-string over the past 30 years. These resources are needed at the undergraduate level, at the graduate level, and at the professional continuing education level.

References

Benner, P. (1984). *From novice to expert: Excellence and power in clinical nursing practice*. Menlo Park, CA: Addison-Wesley.

Benner, P., & Tanner, C. (1987). Clinical judgment: How expert nurses use intuition. *American Journal of Nursing, 87*(1), 23-31.

Benner, P., & Wrubel, J. (1989). *The primacy of caring, stress and coping in health and illness*. Menlo Park, CA: Addison-Wesley.

Borgmann, A. (1984). *Technology and the character of contemporary life*. Chicago: University of Chicago Press.

Bourdieu (1977). *Outline of a theory of practice*. New York: Cambridge University Press.

Collins, H. M. (1985). *Changing order: Replication and induction in scientific practice*. Sage.

Dreyfus, H. L. (1979). *What computers can't do*. New York: Harper & Row.

Dreyfus, H. L. (in press). *Being-in-the-world: A commentary on being and time division I*. Cambridge, MA: MIT Press.

Dreyfus, H. L., & Dreyfus, S. E. (1986). *Mind over machine*. New York: The Free Press.

Heidegger, M. (1982). *The basic problems of phenomenology*. (rev. ed.) (A. A. Hofstadter, Trans.) Bloomington, IN: Indiana University Press.

Kleinman, A., Eisenberg, L., & Good, B. (1978). Culture, illness and care: Clinical lessons from anthropologic and cross cultural research. *Annals of Internal Medicine, 88,* 251.

Lave, J. (1988). *Cognition in practice*. New York: Cambridge University Press.

Lock, M., & Gordon, D. (1988). *Biomedicine examined*. Boston: Kluwer.

Lynaugh, J., & Fagin, C. (1988). Nursing comes of age. *IMAGE: Journal of Nursing Scholarship, 20,* 4.

MacIntyre, A. (1981). *After virtue*. Notre Dame, IN: University of Notre Dame Press.

March, J. G. (1976). The technology of foolishness. In ambiguity and choice in organizations. *Universitetsforlaget,* 69-81.

Menzies, I. (1960). A case study in the functioning of social systems as a defence against anxiety: A report of a study of the nursing service of a general hospital. *Human Relations, 13,* 2.

Merleau-Ponty, M. (1962). *Phenomenology of perception*. (C. Smith, Trans.). London: Routledge and Kegan Paul.

Polanyi, M. (1958). *Personal knowledge*. Chicago: University of Chicago Press.

Suchman, L. A. (1987). *Plans and situated actions, the problem of human-machine communication*. Cambridge, England: Cambridge University Press.

Tripp-Reimer, T. (1984). Reconceptualizing the construct of health: Integrating emic and etic perspectives. *Research in Nursing and Health, 7*(2), 101-109.

Trends and Possibilities in Baccalaureate Nursing Programs

Patricia Moccia

Any discussion on the trends and possibilities in baccalaureate nursing programs is explored most comprehensively within two larger contexts: trends and possibilities in undergraduate education and trends and possibilities in professional education. Once studied, these larger contexts then establish the universe within which our particular concerns can be approached.

Additional factors must be considered, however, when the need for and the integration of critical care content and clinical care experiences in baccalaureate nursing curricula are discussed. The nature of critical care nursing, focused as it is on human responses to life-threatening problems, demands the attention specific to discussions of such fundamental import and deeply profound implications as those that emanate from the distinction between being and nonbeing. This, then, is not just a general discussion of education for practice of a specialty (although it is that). It also pays attention to the special nature of the specialty.

The argument advanced here is that given the trends in both higher and professional education, several unanticipated and untoward effects on (1) both the profession and individual nurses and (2) both the health care delivery system and individual patients would occur if these two AACN position statements (AACN, 1984, 1987) were implemented. First, we would isolate students and faculty further from mainstream educational experiences and, in turn, from access to society's positions of influence. Second, our graduates would be less prepared than they are now to meet society's health care needs. This in turn, would lead to a progressive devaluation of the nursing profession. Third, we would contribute to the further dehumanization of patients who come to the various settings within our delivery systems for assistance with life-threatening problems.

While I have no doubt that we can do what these two position statements recommend, the question we need to consider and discuss is, At what costs to those involved? Several alternative recommendations would preserve what I understand to be the intent of AACN's positions.

Trends in Higher Education

Both higher and professional education continue, for the most part, with philosophies, structures, and processes developed and established in a time vastly different from now. Although a significant educational reform movement occurred throughout the 1960s and the early 1970s, its impact was limited and circumscribed in higher education and barely felt in professional education (Ravich, 1983, Apple, 1982). Now the legitimacy of those small advances is being questioned by educational conservatives and progressives alike, and the advances themselves are compromised by economic imperatives that allow little room for the humanistic commitment that characterized the reforms in the first place (Association of American Colleges, 1985; Bennett, 1984).

If educators are to succeed in their mission of preparing an enlightened citizenry for full participation in the community, they obviously must adjust their institutions and their activities to several recent trends that have altered the fundamental nature of the society within which students and faculty members live. First, educators must recognize that we are in the midst of a cycle of increasing alienation and isolation as the community and commitment necessary for a successful *public* have been undermined by an individualistic private sphere. Furthermore, the isolating experiences of individuals in this private sphere are, in turn, compounded by an isolating and alienating community (Bellah, 1985). Second, there are obvious implications for higher education as the composition and expectations of our student populations match those of the general populations; that is, as the aggregate "we" grows older and becomes increasingly diverse. Third, if it is to be an agent of change, higher education must find some way to accommodate the collapse of the middle class and the widening gap between the poor and the wealthy. Fourth, if higher education is to be financially viable, it must meet the challenges that accompany changes in the government's financial support and assistance of students and institutions.

In addition, higher education necessarily must move toward a fuller integration of the scientific discoveries of the last 25 years. In all its aspects, for example, and not just in its science departments, higher education needs to address the implications of the conceptual revolution in physics that now would have us characterize natural phenomena as complex, irreversibly fluctuating, and random rather than as ordered and predictable (Prigogine & Stengers, 1984); or those discoveries in neurophysics that lead us to understand the holographic, rather than particularistic, nature of human phenomena (Bohm, 1980); or the discoveries in biogenetics that call into question all we have believed before about the distinctions between life and death (Callahan, 1986).

One of the most significant factors in revolutionizing our educational culture might well be a function of what educators have learned from the feminist approaches to science and inquiry developed in the last decades. Fundamental and traditionally asked questions about the nature of science, epistemology, method, and values all are answered differently from a feminist perspective (Blair, 1986, Harding, 1986). In addition, once it is acknowledged, as feminist social scientists would have us do, that women have been "hidden from history," the discovery of their experiences becomes a critical element in developing a new and fuller understanding of our lives (Lerner, 1979). If it is true, as feminist historian Gerda Lerner suggests, that "all of history is to be rewritten" from a feminist perspective, then certainly higher education also will have to reorder itself.

The synergistic impact of these social, scientific, historical and philosophical changes challenges many of the basic assumptions of our educational systems. The nature of our reality is being questioned: Is it unfolding or being created anew each day? The nature of the relationship between people and the physical environment is being rethought: Can it continue to be exploitative rather than empathetic? The nature of the relationships among people has become a puzzle: Is it healthier for individuals and communities to differentiate more sharply, search for their common interests, or somehow manage to do both simultaneously?

In short, a new world view has emerged and continues to do so while educators are caught up in reproducing the old one.

Trends in Professional Education

In addition, to the challenges facing higher education in general, professional education has particular changes with which to contend. The development of the United States from a multinational to an international economy, from an industrial to a service base, and from a blue-collar to a white- and pink-collar work force has implications for the professional and technical sector that have not been addressed yet by education in any systematic way. Furthermore, the professions' claim to specialized and esoteric knowledge has been weakened by technologic advances that make information readily available to anyone who has access to a computer.

Many analysts suggest that the issues go much deeper as the professions find themselves in a "crisis of confidence and legitimacy" (Schon, 1982, p.11). Donald A. Schon, for example, writes in *The Reflective Practitioner* that practitioners find themselves "embroiled in conflicts of values, goals, purposes, and interests" (Schon, 1982, p. 17). He presents the current situation as one in which the old ways of professional education leave the practitioner ill-prepared to work as he or she faces conditions that Schon describes as "complex, uncertain, unstable, unique and laden with value conflicts." (Schon, 1982, pg.18).

This crisis of legitimacy is exacerbated further by the rising costs of professional education for both students and institutions. An increasingly elite professional stratum is created as its members are drawn more and more from the upper middle classes who are able to afford the tuition or to obtain whatever loans might be necessary to attend school (Butter, 1987). Separated by experience from the lives of most of the population and by the need to recoup personal investment from nonprofitable services, professionals are retreating into self-interested activities and away from activities committed to the public interest and the common good (Callahan, 1987). Institutions with responsibilities to existing faculties are faced with resolving the inevitable choice of allocating constricted resources either to programs that reflect existing specialties or to those that respond to emerging needs (Cramton, 1986).

The combined toll of the professions' internal problems and the external lure of more lucrative and less value-conflicted careers can be seen in the declining numbers of applicants for such previously coveted positions as places in medical schools (Iglehart, 1986). In addition, the models for professional education and professional conduct, developed in the early part of the 20th century, increasingly are ill-suited for today's concerns. Although new ways have not been developed, yet most professional disciplines have undertaken serious studies of how things might be otherwise. Even medicine has come to question whether current methods are preparing physicians for a quickly vanishing past and whether the health care provider of the future would be educated more appropriately through programs that emphasize the humanities, social responsibility, managed care, ambulatory care, and community service (Ebert & Ginzberg, 1988, Rogers, in press).

Trends and Possibilities in Nursing Education

Although current and future issues facing nursing education parallel those for higher and professional education in general, some are particular to the situation in which nursing finds itself after a century of progress. The challenge of how to educate nurses for practice within current structures is compounded by several trends. First, nursing students are traditionally from the working and lower-middle classes (Butter, 1987) and therefore are unlikely to have the vast reserves of either time or money that are needed for prolonged educational preparation. Second, even if subsidies were available to either institutions or individuals, comparable rates of return for such an investment as measured in lifelong earnings (Butter, 1987) argue against nursing as a career choice. Third, the emerging public ethos is decidedly unsympathetic to public service (Reamer, 1987). Fourth, if pay scales were adjusted upward to a minimum of comparable worth standards (Youngkin, 1985), the aggregate costs would overwhelm the industry as it presently is structured and financed.

In addition, certain trends in the development of nursing science must be included in our discussion. Twenty-five years ago, questions in the nursing literature debated whether nursing was a science and whether theory development was essential for the profession's advance (Moccia, 1985). Today, those questions put to rest; nurse researchers and practitioners are discussing what *kind* of knowledge — empirical, aesthetic, personal, or ethical — is needed for a theoretically sound nursing practice (Carper, 1978). Today, nurses are learning, discovering, and developing new ways to search for this knowledge — philosophically, historically, phenomenologically, and dialectically — through social and feminist analyses and by applying the critical theoretical approach and refining empirical-analytical methods (Chinn, 1986). The questions emerging from the intensity of this activity over the last 25 years place nurses in the middle of those scientists who are reexamining prevailing world views, existing definitions of science, and current agreements as to what constitutes legitimate knowledge and the ways to obtain it.

In contrast to earlier ambiguities about nursing's focus, today's literature reflects a soundly established metaparadigm that embraces the concepts of people, nursing, health, and the environment (Fawcett, 1984). Our understanding of these concepts has been expanded and deepened so much by nursing scholarship that they are often qualitatively different phenomena than once described. Humans, for example, once defined as bio-psycho-social organisms became bio-psycho-social-cultural-spiritual-(etc.) beings and then holistic phenomena (Meleis, 1985). The definition of health has been transformed from "the absence of disease" to a polar position on the "health-illness continuum" to Newman's idea that health is a "process of expanding consciousness" in which the implicate order is made explicit (Newman, 1986). The concept of the environment, the least developed until recently, is being reconceptualized by some to focus on society's social-political and economic structures, human, social relations, and everyday life in order to inform nursing theory and practice more productively (Chopoorian).

Although these concepts and the relationships among them have been developed and extended significantly by nursing scholarship and research, they usually have added to, rather than replaced, more traditional medical and social sciences in nursing curricula. We are now at the point of discussing how curricula might change to reflect all these trends (Curriculum Revolution, Mandate for Change, 1988). We are discussing such topics as the moral context for education, the practice mandate, a reconsideration of the Tyler model of curriculum development, new teaching-learning relationships, new student populations, how to educate students for home and long-term care, and how to use adjunct faculty.

Finally, and perhaps most significantly, if the Washington axiom, "As goes Medicare, so goes health care," prevails, a recent piece of federal legislation might be the most determining of all these factors for how nursing education develops. Bentsen and Chafee, with the support of Dole, sponsored an initiative that provides funding, via Medicare pass-through, for five demonstration projects in hospitals that have clinical training for graduate nursing students. Signed into law by President Reagan on November 11, 1988, the Bensten-Chafee bill establishes a precedent for nursing education and, depending on how the demonstration projects fare, the financial incentive for specialization at the graduate level. This is the context within which AACN's position statements will be received and evaluated by nursing colleagues.

Untoward Effects

On first glance, few responsible educators could argue with either of the AACN position statements on integration of critical care content and clinical experiences in baccalaureate nursing curricula.

Although the intent to ensure the availability of competent practitioners for increasingly complex patient problems is obviously an appropriate and responsible position, difficulties exist in some of the assumptions that underlie the proposed strategies. In an ironic pair of contradictions, the position statements seem to assume that undergraduate education is infinitely malleable and that the structure of future delivery systems will remain relatively intact. Most analyses suggest exactly the opposite for each of the arenas. By not accounting for the limits of undergraduate education or the transformation of the delivery system, the position statements lead us away from where I think we would like to be.

First, we would isolate undergraduate students and faculty members further, from mainstream educational experiences and, in turn, from access to society's positions of influence. Put most simply, the traditional 128-credit undergraduate program has just so much elasticity. Nursing curricula already are stretched to the snapping point by educators' attempts to integrate all we have urged each other to include in our undergraduate programs: legal, ethical, cultural, and historical aspects of our profession; research and nursing science; the principles and skills of communication and leadership; theories of organizational behavior, fiscal management, and marketing; public policy, political advocacy, and social responsibility; home care and gerontology — to name just a few. This superabundance of content has just about transformed most nursing courses into overviews and surveys rather than the detailed studies expected of those who major in an area. Nursing students barely are introduced to ideas, rather than provided with the time and opportunities for in-depth study. Graduate nurses, then, begin their careers with only the most superficial of understanding about their profession and about their practice.

Coupled with the educational demands of this explosion of theoretical knowledge are the equally overwhelming increases in the acuity and complexity of patient problems, as AACN acknowledges in the first "whereas" of the 1987 position statement. It follows that the amount of specific preparation time for clinical experiences such as those proposed will continue to increase also. The amount of time needed for faculty members to maintain their clinical expertise and for students to perfect increasingly complex and sophisticated skills will increase too.

For students to meet successfully even the barest minimum of standards in each of these areas, other parts of their lives necessarily will be compromised. Students can learn to cope with these tandem demands by lowering their own expectations and standards and accepting "just getting by" by withdrawing from all social, familial and community interactions for the course of their studies; by electing to meet liberal arts requirements with "gut" courses; by delaying their pursuit of other interests and developing other talents; or by combining all these strategies. However, no matter what choice they make, one of the most basic arguments for baccalaureate education for nurses will have been negated, namely, that nurses should be educated comprehensively within institutions of higher learning in order that they might develop their potential fully as leaders in society. An issue for us to address and resolve is that as students (and faculty members) live through the reality of incorporating critical care content and direct clinical experiences in baccalaureate nursing curricula, they most likely will do so in increasing isolation from students in other disciplines and fields, in patterns that increasingly will resemble nurses' training.

Second, our graduates would be even less prepared than they are now to meet society's health care needs. This, which, in turn, would lead to a progressive devaluation of the nursing profession. Demographic, economic, and technological factors are driving health care away from tertiary inpatient care systems and are changing the nature of those systems that are managing to survive as the current changes in production, financing, and organization of services run their course. Changes in payer systems are transforming the culture of health care into a managed care environment. In addition, as the payers drive down the demand for acute care services, advances in science and technology, such as laser surgery, will contribute to a decrease in the number of invasive procedures performed, and with that further decrease the demand for inpatient services. Still further changes are emerging now as the population grows older, as our social fabric becomes increasingly torn and tattered, and as the health needs of our communities demand more comprehensive care — whether institution or community based.

Nurse educators surely can succeed in the task of integrating critical care content and clinical experiences into the baccalaureate curricula. However, several questions arise: Who will be accountable for programs that graduate students who have outmoded and obsolete skills? Where will these graduates find employment? Who will answer their questions about the discrepancies between their education for autonomous professional practice and their experiences in an increasingly bureaucratic, technically dominated system? How and where will they express their frustration and sense of betrayal at an education that prepared them for the past rather than the present and the future? Where and how will they reenter the educational system? How have they been prepared to continue their education?

Third, we would contribute to the further dehumanization of patients who come to the various settings within our delivery systems for assistance with life-threatening problems. The particular nature of critical care nursing as a specialty calls for a particular set of questions to be addressed: Is it possible for a beginning practitioner to provide the extent of the biopsychosocial care that can be anticipated as being needed by patients with life-threatening problems? Is it possible to educate beginning practitioners in the breadth and depth of what it means for individuals and their friends and families to face the possibility of death and dying? Is it possible to educate beginning practitioners to manage the comprehensive care that such patients need?

Given the increasing complexity of patients' problems and the decreasing specialization possible within higher and professional education, I think not. As the two trends continue in their opposite directions, it becomes increasingly unlikely that beginning practitioners will have the knowledge, skill, professional sophistication, or personal maturity to provide critically ill patients with comprehensive nursing care. Before implementing the resolutions in these position statements, we need to consider seriously (1) whether we will be asking beginning practitioners to do the impossible and (2) what will be the personal toll on nurses when they fail to meet these unrealistic expectations.

Consider this beginning practitioner we send to the patient's bedside and the influence that this person has on the nurse-patient interaction. Consider, if it brings it closer to home, the beginning practitioner we will be sending to the bedside of a friend or family member and the kind of interaction that will occur. Given the constraints of the undergraduate curriculum and the demands of the critical care setting, the nurse will be a superb technician, a well-rounded generalist, or some hybrid of the two who accomplished the merger at the sacrifice of personal development. And, the interaction between this nurse and the patient will reflect the choices the nurse made to survive and succeed in both academia and practice. In any case, the interaction will be less than a fully integrated one and, therefore, will potentiate the process of dehumanization that accompanies all interactions with a bureaucratic delivery system and that is even more pronounced when advanced technology is introduced.

Before we move to implement the resolutions of either of the position statements, I urge us to reconsider the resolutions in light of (1) the trends in higher and professional education that direct our programs and curricula away from specialization and toward a more generalist approach and (2) the trends in the delivery system that direct the production, organization, and financing of services away from tertiary, acute care toward a managed care system at the primary and secondary level.

Recommendations for Future Study

For purposes of discussion, I suggest that we assume the feasibility, of the following recommendations:

1. Reform undergraduate nursing education. Move toward an approach to learning that includes a closer and fuller integration of theory-practice-research activities, a more anthropological approach to learning about the health and humanity of our populations, and the embrace of a teacher-apprentice model, and move away from an approach that includes discrete disciplines and subject matter, an overdependence on the needs of the current delivery system as determinants of curricula and a dominant-submissive teacher-student relationship.
2. Reform undergraduate education for all health care providers. Move toward the preparation of a generalist, who will receive a truly interdisciplinary education, be granted a newly created degree (bachelor's in health and human sciences?), and be expected to go on to graduate studies.
3. Reform graduate nursing education as specialist preparation, at both the master's and postmaster's level. Move toward distinct, but not necessarily mutually exclusive, careers as clinicians, researchers, teachers, and administrators, with faculty members prepared as specialists and schools, programs, and curricula developed as specialty centers.

References

Among the contemporary critiques: Association of American Colleges. (1985). *Integrity in the college curriculum: A report to the academic community*. Washington, D.C.; Bennett, W. J. (1984). To reclaim a legacy: A report on the humanities in higher education. Washington, D.C.: National Endowment for the Humanities; & Ravitch, D. (1983). *The troubled crusade: American education 1945-1980*. New York: Basic Books.

Among the feminists: Bleir, R. (Ed). (1986). *Feminist approaches to science*. New York: Pegamon Press; & S. Harding, (1986). The Science Question in Feminism. Ithaca: Cornell University Press.

Among the progressive reformists: Apple, M. W. (1982). *Education and power*. Boston: Ark; Bowles, S. & Gintis H. (1976). Schooling in capitalist America. New York: Basic Books; & Freire, P. (1973). *Education for critical consciousness*. New York: Seabury Press.

Bellah, R., et al. (1985). *Habits of the heart. Individualism and commitment in American life*. New York: Harper & Row.

Bohm, D. (1980). *Wholeness and the implicate order*. London: Ark Paperbacks.
Butter, I., et al. (1987). Gender hierarchies in the health labor force. *International Journal of Health Services, 17*(1), 133-149.
Callahan, D. (February 1986). How technology is reframing the abortion debate. *Hastings Center Report, 16*(1), 33-42.
Callahan, D. (February, 1987). Introduction to the public duties of the professions. *Hastings Center Reports, Special Supplement, 17*(1).
Carper, B. A. (1978). Fundamental patterns of knowing in nursing. *Advances in Nursing Science, 1*(1), 13-23.
Chinn, P. L. (1986). *Nursing research methodology. Issues and implementation*. Rockville, MD: Aspen.
Chopoorian, T. Reconceptualizing the Environment. In Moccia, P. (1985). *New approaches to theory development*. New York: National League for Nursing.
Cramton, R. C. (Fall 1986). Lessons for medicine from legal education. *Health Affairs, 5* (3), 34-45.
Curriculum revolution: Mandate for change. (1988). New York: National League for Nursing.
Ebert, R. H. & Ginzberg, E. (1988). The reform of medical education. *Health Affairs*, Special Supplement, 5-38.
Fawcett, J. (1984). The metaparadigm of nursing: Present status and future refinement. *Image, 16,* 3.
Iglehart, J. K. (Fall 1986). Update. From physician shortage to patient shortage: The uncertain future of medical practice. *Health Affairs, 5*(3), 142-151.
Lerner, G. (1979). *The majority finds its past. Placing women in history*. New York: Oxford University Press.
Meleis, A. (1985). Theory development and domain concepts. In Moccia, P. *New approaches to theory development*. New York: National League for Nursing.
Moccia, P.(1985). *New approaches to theory development*. New York: National League for Nursing.
Newman, M. A. (1986). *Health as expanding consciousness*. St. Louis: C. V. Mosby.
Prigogine, I. & Stengers, I. (1984). *Order out of chaos*. Toronto: Bantam Books.
Reamer, F. (February 1987). Social work: Calling or career? *Hastings Center Reports*, Special Supplement, 17(1), 14-15.
Rogers, D. E. (In press). Clinical education and the doctor of tomorrow. In Gastel, B. & Rogers, D. E. (Eds.) Adapting clinical medical education to the needs of today and tomorrow. New York: The New York Academy of Medicine.
Schon, D. A. (1982). *The reflective practitioner*. New York: Basic Books.
Youngkin, E. Q. (January-February 1985). Comparable worth: Alternatives to litigation and legislation. *Nursing Economics, 3,* 38-43.

Response to Benner and Moccia: An Educator's Response

Ellen B. Rudy

It is a pleasure to be given the opportunity to respond to the papers by Drs. Benner and Moccia. I read somewhere in the program description that the conference participants would be "opinion leaders" in nursing. If there is one thing you can count on from me, it is to have an opinion.

Actually, I asked to be a panel member at this conference. The Case Western Reserve University School of Nursing is reinitiating its baccalaureate of nursing program, and it will have a focus on acute and critical care nursing. The program will be the usual 4 academic years, but students will begin clinical experience the first semester, with increasing time each year, so that in their last year, students will spend 3 days each week in acute and critical care settings.

The program obviously will have the usual content and clinical experience in maternity, pediatric, psychiatric, community health, and medical-surgical nursing. Our attempt will be to provide these experiences whenever possible with a focus on acute care. For example, community health nursing will cover the usual preventive and health promotion programs, but it also will include some time in home health care agencies. Students will help take care of patients who are on ventilators or receiving total parenteral nutrition; change dressings; and deal with the concomitant problems of family coping, family crisis, and family cost.

Perhaps the most unusual feature of this baccalaureate program is that we have formed a consortium that includes the Francis Payne

Bolton School of Nursing and three major hospitals in Cleveland: the Cleveland Clinic, Cleveland MetroHealth Medical Center, and University Hospitals of Cleveland. Each hospital will identify approximately 34 students each year whom they will support by providing 50% tuition, clinical mentors, and summer employment. This support will be for all 4 years of this program. After graduation, the student will be required to work at the sponsoring hospital for 2 years.

I mention this program only because it is different, both in clinical focus and in the collaboration between the School of Nursing and the hospitals. Other baccalaureate programs have focused on primary care, with practitioner skills or distributive care (when "episodic" and "distributive" were the buzz words) and so forth, but it has not been the trend in nursing education in the past 20 years to focus attention on the hospitalized patient and the patient's family. The fact that I support such a program tells you what my biases are.

My comments on the papers that have been presented will be organized as follows: First I want to highlight and make more explicit — or less invisible — the major themes that I believe Dr. Benner's paper provided. Next, I want to use this, along with my own experience, to challenge some of the statements in Dr. Moccia's paper. And, finally, I want to end with my own thoughts on the inclusion of critical care nursing in the baccalaureate curriculum.

Major Themes

Let me begin with Dr. Benner's comments. Critical care nursing, the gestalt of this practice, indeed has developed within the ranks of nursing with little visibility, few resources, and little recognition. Although this is true for the most part, the point Dr. Benner *did not* make is the amazing appeal of critical care nursing to practicing nurses. Critical care nursing as a specialty within nursing has bloomed. The fact that AACN has more than 60,000 members as the largest nursing specialty organization is a fairly good indication that *within* the ranks of nursing, critical care is visible.

I think that two major movements within nursing, not in academic nursing education until recently, but within the ranks of *nurses*, have had a profound effect on our status, our power, and *our access to patients*. They are the development of critical care nursing and nurse practitioner programs. To quote Dr. Benner, we now have "illegitimate authority, indirect power, and a pattern of status inequity". Nonetheless, this is an improvement compared with other areas in which nurses practice, in which they often have less authority, less power, and lower status, for example the nurse in a general medical-surgical division.

Dr. Benner's paper itself was full of the richness that she ascribes to knowledge imbedded within the critical care clinician. It is, therefore, not always easy to boil down and crystalize in a few sentences. I would highlight two major points.

The first is her comment on technology: "Critical care nurses cannot be reduced to the level of mere technicians even though they must be exquisite technicians." Indeed, health care today means technology; without an understanding of and skill with technology, the nurse, especially the student nurse, cannot move on to the caring.

Faculty members in undergraduate nursing programs have known this for eons. A student nurse cannot comfort a crying child who is being fed via a tube until the nurse is able to manipulate the equipment used for tube feeding. The same is true for intravenous medications. I have had students so frightened and insecure the first time they gave medication by using the intravenous "piggy back" method that I honestly think if I had asked the color and sex of the patient after the medication had been given, the students would not have been able to tell me. Their entire "being" was focused on the needle, the tubing and the intravenous bag.

Technology is a part of nursing. Thus, to become comfortable and competent requires repeated clinical exposure to technology. To become caring requires a measure of comfort and competence with technology so that technology no longer is the focus of care, so that the patient becomes the focus.

I concur with Dr. Benner that "nurses traditionally had a strong commitment to rehabilitation, recovery, community health care and health promotion." This so-called general focus inappropriately has been equated with low technology. The technical skills required in primary care and community care no longer allow such differentiation, simply because of equipment and machines required to provide the care. Technology is not the differentiation from a general focus to a specialty focus. To ignore technology and the need for technical skills or to relegate these to acute care only is to be outdated and limited in our abilities.

The second point made by Dr. Benner that I would like to highlight is her recognition of the wealth of invisible and poorly articulated knowledge that these clinicians discover, use, and pass on to one another. The problem, of course, is that it is not enough to recognize this knowledge — if it is knowledge and not just hunches or ritual — it needs testing and dissemination. The collaboration between practice and education could facilitate this process. Academic faculty members need to do research and publish, and critical care clinicians could provide the ideas and the access to patients and be active members in this knowledge-building process. This knowledge should not be allowed to remain invisible and institution specific. Instead, if interventions really work, they should be submitted to testing and shared with the outside world.

Challenges

Turning now to Dr. Moccia's comments, which are philosophically different from my own, I want to begin with our points of agreement. I agree, for the most part, with her overview on the trends in higher education and in professional education. Higher education must take care that it does not become restricted to the privileged few, and indeed a new world view is emerging that poses many new questions, such as whether a frozen embryo is, in fact, life and can inherit from an estate.

Dr. Moccia's argument that nursing students should have the time and opportunity to be a part of educational life that examines these and many broader and more complicated questions reminds me of the beautifully articulated argument of Schlotfeldt (1978) who proposed that nurses should receive professional education *after* they had earned an undergraduate degree in a program in which they could be part of the mainstream educational system. This concept, the doctorate in nursing as the first professional degree earned after a baccalaureate degree, is a concept I continue to believe in, but it is one that the nursing profession has not embraced, and one that appears more difficult to put into operation in light of the cyclical nursing shortages.

Therefore, at times I too lament the rigor of the nursing curriculum, which takes its toll on our students. I find, however, when I burrow out of my self-absorbed maze, that students in other professions, such as architecture, optometry, and engineering, are also hard at work for long hours and often at the expense of family and social activities.

Now to those points with which I take exception. Nursing curricula indeed are stretched to the snapping point because of the tendency to add new content on gerontology, ethics, and so forth, but without ever deleting old content. Her comment that graduates all too often begin their careers with only the most superficial understanding about their profession and about their practice is also true. Faculty members allow that to happen.

I suggest to you that faculty members must face the dilemmas of (1) what logically belongs in an undergraduate curriculum and (2) how do we make sure that the knowledge and skills required to be a professional nurse are acquired before graduation. Undergraduate education must not be recall and regurgitation. We must teach students how to learn, how to acquire the knowledge necessary for nursing *now*, and how to use this process of learning for teaching themselves after graduation — the old cliche of life-long learning. I see this process at the graduate level, but rarely at the undergraduate level, of teaching students how to teach themselves. How many of our baccalaureate graduates never have a professional journal come into their homes?

Teaching critical care content and having clinical experience in critical care will do exactly the opposite from what Dr. Moccia claims. A critical care environment provides unlimited opportunities for concentrated teaching. A new graduate can learn about technologies, crisis management, mechanisms for reduction of anxiety, family coping, ethical dilemmas, and the importance of touch and of talking to the very ill — all this before 11 a.m. My point is, of course, that this cannot be done all at once, but a critical care clinical experience provides the instructor many opportunities for teaching and the students many opportunities for gaining that elusive confidence students are expected to attain.

When I taught critical care to undergraduates, I never had to worry about whether I would have the experiences the students needed. There were always more things to learn than time to learn them. Where better to address death and dying and health promotion than with a 40-year old man who had had a massive heart attack and was in cardiogenic shock? Students who smoked could not help but examine themselves after our clinical conference. Where better to help students examine the difference in the professional and personal conflict faced in gaining a Do Not Resuscitate order for a patient with acquired immune deficiency syndrome.

I think that a curriculum that does not include a critical care clinical experience (and I do not mean observation) is outmoded and obsolete and that students in such a program are receiving less than a quality education. It is true that the current emphasis on acute care may *change* and that faculty members must be willing to adjust the curriculum accordingly, but I cannot tell you how tired I am of hearing that nursing is moving out of acute care facilities.

In 1923, the Goldmark Report (Winslow et al., 1923) spoke to the need for public health nurses to improve the health of mothers and children. Baccalaureate schools of nursing added public health nursing to the curriculum to prepare students for nursing in the community and predicted less need for hospital nurses. In the 1970's Lysaught coined the terms "episodic" and "distributive" care. Episodic care was hospital care and short-term, and thus nurses should prepare themselves for the *real* need, distributive care. In 1983, with the implementation of prospective payment, the prediction was that patients would be kept out of hospitals and discharged quickly so that nurses would move out of the hospital.

The predictions of all these reports have been correct to a degree, but the facts are that 70% of all nurses in the work force work in hospitals. The Secretary's Commission on Nursing (1988), which listened to testimony and made recommendations on the nursing shortage, criticized schools of nursing for the fewer and fewer hours dedicated to clinical learning experiences. Finally, in a survey by NLN of recent graduates (Rosenfeld, 1988), most of whom are working in hospitals, more than one quarter were dissatisfied with their clinical preparation on graduation.

Our learning laboratory is the setting in which the patients receive nursing. The critical care setting offers a concentrated and rich laboratory for teaching nursing skills and professional decision making. Expert faculty members can take advantage of this laboratory to teach a wide variety of nursing content.

This exposure to high technology and high human needs is a good foundation for learning to (1) provide home care for the elderly who are bedridden; (2) care for the ventilator-dependent teenager or the high-risk maternity patient; (3) help families deal with early fetal loss; or (4) question the wisdom of resource allocations that neglect the poor and the elderly.

Having said all this, let me echo my agreement with Dr. Hawken that it is inappropriate for the NLN to require an experience in critical care nursing. The accreditation criteria for the league have been improved greatly over the years and now require primarily that the curriculum be organized and explicated logically and that it be a product that is determined by the school's faculty. Such a format permits evolution and appropriate change as the health care industry changes and the educational needs of nursing change.

Suggestions

As you can tell from these papers and the responses, opinions are diverse and at times in direct conflict. I have two suggestions to make. First, I suggest AACN find individuals who understand the value of critical care clinical experiences and have these individuals infiltrate various faculty groups throughout the United States. I have been impressed immensely with how much influence one committed faculty member can have on a school's curriculum.

Second, I think that the key to having good critical care experiences for undergraduate students is to have a good practice-education relationship. This means a relationship in which faculty members and students are welcomed in the clinical setting and in which faculty members are well prepared and maintain their clinical expertise so that staff nurses have confidence in their ability to handle the critically ill patient.

References

Lysaught, J. P. (1970). *An abstract for action*. New York: McGraw-Hill.

Rosenfeld, P. (1988). *Newly licensed nurses: Study presentation*. New York: National League for Nursing.

Schlotfeldt, R. M. (1978). The professional doctorate: Rationale and characteristics. *Nursing Outlook, 26,* 302, 311.

Secretary's Commission on Nursing (1988). *Final report* (Vol. 1). Washington, DC: Department of Health and Human Services.

Winslow, C. E. A., et al., (1923). *Nursing and nursing education in the United States*. New York: MacMillan.

Response to Benner and Moccia: An Educator's Response

Jeanette Lancaster

I appreciate the opportunity to respond to two interesting and provocative papers. The papers are quite different from each other and clearly reflect the interests and expertise of the authors.

Dr. Benner pointed out that expert, intensive critical care nursing is only 30 years old, and that as a specialty area of nursing, it is largely invisible. In the study she and her colleagues are conducting on intensive care nursing practice, their preliminary analysis has identified nine causes of invisibility. As I read the description of these nine causes, I first saw them not so much as examples of invisibility but as testimony to the caring and sophisticated decision making, clinical judgment, and creativity that are evidenced by critical care nurses.

The facts necessary to practice effectively in this nursing specialty are enormous, and the blending of precise knowledge (in the presence of life-threatening health problems and urgency related to time) and the need to maintain vital human contact through touch and voice is a significant challenge. I think we would agree with Dr. Benner that critical care nurses need to be expert technicians and also must be immensely caring. The challenge to show caring to patients and their families is substantial. Health status can change rapidly, and the need for decisions about how to use precious minutes are ever-present.

Many would agree that American society values cure more than care. We reflect our values in such concrete ways as reimbursement.

Physicians and other healers earn considerably more than nurses and other members of the health care team who primarily are charged with providing care designed to reinforce and often actually implement the curative functions. I never have been convinced that cure and care must be separate nor that they should be mutually exclusive. Each of us can think of numerous instances in which it takes no additional time to give assistance designed to cure that also reflects caring rather than to focus exclusively on cure with little or no attention to caring. Some nurses, indeed persons in all aspects of life, seem to care intuitively for others. They recognize silent, nonverbal cues that reflect needs, and they respond accordingly. Other nurses who are not by nature as sensitive, perceptive, and caring can be taught how to recognize cues and how to care enough to respond to those cues.

I agree with Dr. Benner that within our undergraduate programs we can teach our students to observe, to make astute and accurate clinical decisions, and to care enough for patients to respond to the patients' expressed, as well as more covert, needs. I also agree that talking about practice in a critical care setting or observing nurses in this setting for 1 or 2 days is inadequate to fulfill the resolutions for incorporating critical care content into undergraduate education as advocated by the AACN.

Dr. Moccia began by taking exception to the request by AACN that undergraduate programs need to incorporate critical care learning experiences into the curriculum. Her rationale, and logical one, was that currently undergraduate nursing programs are "packed" with content. Clearly, many specialty organizations want students to be given more intense education relative to the specialty's area of interest. Dr. Moccia argued for a general nursing education at the undergraduate level built on a strong foundation in the liberal arts.

Indeed, in the late 1980s, nearly all colleges and universities have implemented new and more extensive general education requirements designed to provide a more integrated and carefully thought-out liberal foundation than we have seen before other than at the declared liberal arts colleges. Traditionally, students have been allowed far more freedom than they currently have in developing their own general education packages. Now universities are becoming prescriptive so that all graduates will be assured of receiving a liberal education base that includes such things as mathematics; English; foreign languages; social, natural, and behavioral sciences; and attention to both Western and Eastern cultures.

I think it is possible, though not necessarily easy, to provide within the undergraduate program a core of general education and both general and selected specialty education. I heartily support Dr.

Moccia's recommendation that the undergraduate nursing program should provide graduates with generalist nursing knowledge and skills. Likewise, I endorse her contention that our approach to learning should include "a closer and fuller integration of theory-practice-research activities." I am not sure such integration requires reform. Many of us would say our schools are already on the right track and perhaps just need a boost in this area. I disagree with Dr. Moccia's second recommendation that we should reform undergraduate education for all health care providers. I am, however, unclear has to how that recommendation fits into the domain of nursing. Seemingly, we have enough to do in our reform, or perhaps refinement, of our own undergraduate and graduate programs without spending too much time on other health professions.

In my opinion and experience, we in education must join as full partners with our colleagues in the practice arena to change our educational programs to meet the request of AACN and to educate caring and competent practitioners. Let me share an example. In 1984, Wright State University entered into a collaborative agreement with Miami Valley Hospital, a 740-bed, private, not-for-profit hospital. We instituted joint programs of nursing research and had joint appointees (the hospital has more than 70 nurses with master's degrees and three with doctorates). Wright State students were given first choice of the hospital's clinical units. Also, the university began appointing hospital staff members to school committees and the hospital appointed university faculty members to hospital committees.

This enterprise began almost simultaneously with the onset of diagnosis-related groups and the need for hospitals to contain costs. Miami Valley Hospital spends considerable money on nurse recruitment and development through an internship in critical care nursing, an extern program, and extensive staff development. One of the hospital's concerns was that it eventually would need to reduce the costs of orientation. Concurrently, with the close of the hospital's diploma program (no others exist in our area), a supply of new graduates with any experience in areas such as critical care, perioperative care, or neonatal intensive care no longer would be available. The university wanted students to have more content and clinical experience in oncology and gerontology than that usually available in the undergraduate curriculum. To realize these dreams, the university and the hospital established a partnership relationship for teaching clinical electives.

In Wright State's nursing program, all students must take one nursing elective course; they may, however, take more than one. The elective course can be totally didactic or a didactic plus a clinical section. Clinical courses in such areas as perioperative or critical care are expensive because of the need for a low student-to-faculty ratio, so these elective courses are taught as a joint education and service venture. Hospital employees participate in both classroom and clinical teaching. Although clinical courses take more time than totally didactic courses, they are popular with students. In the fall of 1988, student enrollment was such that we offered two sections of perioperative nursing. The course was taught by one faculty member, one joint appointee, the director of surgical nursing and, preceptors who volunteered to participate.

We just completed an elective course in critical care nursing. This 10-week course devoted the first 5 weeks to theory and the second 5 to a preceptorship in a critical care unit. The course had seven students and two faculty members. An additional two to three students could have been accommodated inasmuch as each student also was assigned to a preceptor. All the preceptors volunteered to participate and were enthusiastic about the opportunity.

Clinical courses are time-consuming for faculty members, and you may wonder why they willingly would develop such a program. The faculty members say they spend more time teaching a clinical rather than a didactic course because they believe in what they are doing. They find the course energizing, and it also helps them maintain their clinical skills.

The faculty members and I have not found it possible to integrate critical care clinical experience into the basic curriculum because such an integration is a labor-intensive and expensive task. It is difficult to have 10 students in the critical care area at one time. Also, faculty members have found that it takes a lot of time to make all the necessary arrangements for the course. An elective course was more feasible for us than making this specialty content a requirement.

Hence, I speak in favor of a sound general education core, generalist nursing knowledge and experience, and opportunities for specialty practice that fit students' interests and career goals and faculty members' expertise and interests.

Dr. Benner spoke about the need to equip our graduates not only to deal with the technical complexities of critical care but also to cope effectively with the ethical dilemmas and conflicts inherent in this setting. Let me share one more example of how we at Wright State help equip our students to cope with today's complex health care decisions. The schools of medicine and nursing, in conjunction with United Theological Seminary (a Methodist school), offer four interdisciplinary elective courses. Each course has 10 students and one faculty member per school, plus a resource person from each discipline at each class. The courses are ethics from an interprofessional context, living with loss, human abuse, and suicide prevention.

These courses have been highly successful. The nursing and theology students tend to be older than those from medicine and to have had more diverse life experiences. Students who learn to deal with theoretical dilemmas together seemingly have a better foundation for dealing later with real-life experiences. These elective courses offer safe arenas for debate, disagreement, and personal and professional growth.

In summary, I agree with Dr. Benner that our task is to seek the time, place, resources, and (I would add) creativity to teach critical care nursing in concert with the preparation of a well-educated generalist. It can be done!

SECTION 3
Linking Education and Practice

Relative Roles and Responsibilities of Education and Practice

Sheila A. Ryan

The number of beds for critical care reportedly has increased by 14% in the past year. Projections for the next several years suggest an additional increase of up to 30% to 40%. It is estimated that the total number of hospital beds will continue to decline until the number of beds for critical care will be 40% of the total. In addition, the number of admissions per 1,000 patient days will continue to decline, along with patients' length of stay. It is predicted that more than 700, or 10%, of the nation's hospitals will close by 1995 (Wesbury, 1988).

It is no surprise to learn that the vacancies for critical care nurses and the turnover rates are higher than for other sectors of hospital care. These data are compounded by the fact that critical care nurses need specialized experience and knowledge, that most critical care positions are full time and that most time is already spent in direct patient care and cannot be improved by using alternative models of care providers. (Searle, 1988). What this scenario clearly portrays is not a shortage, or lack of supply, but an increasing demand — A health care system that is becoming multiple critical care units.

I congratulate the AACN for proposing that more education be required at the entry and advanced levels of nursing in the field of critical care. It seems to me that this is a turnaround from the "we can do it for less" message of the past two decades.

Future Issues in Health Care

Before we can examine the agenda for practice and education in the critical care delivery system of tomorrow, let me summarize the six major issues of the future in health care. (Amara, 1988). First there will be three major players (and payers): business, government, and the consumer. Business increasingly will demand a cost-squeezed product. Because of the current federal budget deficits, the government will continue to constrain its spending through the 1990s and to regulate what and how much it will pay. Consumers, who are better educated and more sophisticated, will demand more of a role in traditional decision making. They will resist the efforts to have them pay a higher share of increasing costs. The demand for a measurable, quality, and cost-effective product will be heard from all three players.

Second, we have an overcapacity of hospital beds, physicians, and health care personnel in the United States despite the plea that we do not don't have enough. We have 11 health care personnel per patient, compared with 4 per patient in the Canadian system, and 5 or 6 per patient in the British system, systems that have lower costs and higher health care indexes (i.e., mortality and morbidity). The key question is with fewer people, how will we be able to keep up with the demand through the 1990s? Will increased competition — or regulation, as it is perceived by some — continue to increase or decrease the utilization pace per capita population? Can we, in effect, lower demand?

Third, the core of our current system will continue to be one of high intensity, high technology, and high costs. Hospital admissions and length of stay will continue to decline through the late 1990s and possibly rebound because of the aging cohort.

Fourth, even though the elderly are causing great strains in today's marketplace, by 2000 the number of long-term care, home care, community primary, and health promotion support systems will increase, resulting in less technology and less institutional care. The key issue here is, Where will the money come from to build these community linkages? Some say it will be at the cost of the acute care budget and medical care; others say it cannot be.

Fifth, health care costs will continue to go up. Projections indicate a 70% increase between 1985 and 2000. Attempts to minimize spiraling costs have not succeeded in reducing rates of inflation to single digits. All of this means corresponding increases in administration, managed care systems, cost-controlling and cost-constraining efforts, and quality measures in data collection systems in order to justify these increasing costs.

The sixth and last issue is the spiraling increase in technology (i.e., drugs, devices, techniques, computers, and molecular and genetic manipulations). Technology will become more complex, more expensive, and more pervasive, presenting incredibly tough choices about who gets and who pays, and at what costs to others who do not get. Curricula need significant development in the area of technology: its development, models of testing, assessment, evaluation, and cost implications. (Lindeman, 1988) Nursing time and resources dedicated to technology rather than caring need to be evaluated. There is demand for an increase in ethical, moral reasoning, and advocate models of decision support technology.

Suffice it to say that nurses run more miles per shift today than they did 5 years ago; use more medical devices (10,000 new products licensed in 1988 with the U.S. Food and Drug Administration); and handle tubes, products, medications, procedures, and monitors more frequently than before — all products of technology. The central question I will continue to ask is, How do these help in our mission in the healing art of caring? Does intensive care, which I may equate erroneously with environments of intensive, complex, and sophisticated technology, decrease mortality and morbidity? That is to say, are the increased costs worth it qualitatively? To date, no studies have documented this correlation.

As technology increases costs, does caring decline? Is a caring environment essential for technology to make a difference? As technology escalates, are we able to escalate the caring that is needed? Certainly critical care units are not the exclusive settings for technology and increased acuity and intensity. They are perhaps the extreme. As such, they are worthy settings to answer these questions.

Strategies for Dealing with Technology

The following three strategies or responses for dealing with technology in critical care practice may guide our future educational endeavors: The first is keeping up with it. Education needs to find mechanisms to keep nurses informed of new technological devices; help them provide competent care to patients who have medical devices; and develop procedures for quality assessment and evaluation, including better labeling by manufacturers and vendors. There are also alarming safety issues, such as the increase in nosocomial infections that are device related (45%); infections or phlebitis develop in half the patients who have intravascular devices. Nurses are often responsible for providing all the on going continuing education about a device and its use and for all required maintenance and monitoring and infrequently are involved in the design of the device or the selection of vendor products.

Education needs to design a new curriculum that focuses on the development and evaluation of technology. Certainly, principles of how technology works could be prioritized into understanding the principles of fluids, electricity, conductivity, and physics. We have an additional imperative to develop a central repository of device-specific information that would be readily accessible and available on-line in the nursing units.

The second strategy is constraining the use of technology. The premise underlying this discussion is that of ethical and economic considerations and the risk-benefit advantages of technology — that is, who should get the benefits, and at what price? Victor Fuchs labeled this the technological imperative. (Fuchs, 1968). Heaney, 1987, translates this simply:

> We can, therefore we must. We each know from experience that everything possible simply cannot be synonymous with the best. We are each all too familiar with many heroic interventions that occur at the end of life, ranging from the initiation of dialysis in permanently comatose patients, multicardiovascular resuscitation in the final week of life of people dying of multiple myeloma — the examples are too numerous and too painful to recount. Such unrestrained use of technology produces almost uniformly bad results — increased suffering for all, and huge costs that strain the health care financing system. (p. 3)

The technological imperative is operative not only in desperate situations, so says Heaney, but whenever there is any opportunity to intervene, either diagnostically or therapeutically:

> Uncomfortable as it may be to do so, we need to examine our infatuation with technical fixes, examine what it is we value, what we think more and less important, and where we chose to put our emphasis and resources. Will it be razzle-dazzle, medical miracles, dramatic saves, therapeutic virtuosity, great efforts expended to solve the problems of a very few? Or will it be elevating the health status of the many, dealing with the problems of the elderly and the poor? Improving the quality of life for those whom the system can't cure, preventing what we know how to prevent? (p. 3)

Let me be clear about my purpose. I am not against technology. I simply am concerned that we control it: it seems quite certain that if we do not, it will control us. In fact, we need to examine the situations systematically whenever we embark on technological courses of action that predictably have bad outcomes or will cause needless suffering. There are always times, and we know them, when doing less than everything possible is clearly the best strategy. It can be shown graphically that palliative and supportive therapies have a predictable distribution of outcomes, not all good, and not all bad; most are somewhere in the middle. However, the frequency of good outcomes that occur as a result of definitive interventions is lower than the frequency of the worst of outcomes (Heaney, 1987).

Virtually all medical interventions have good and bad effects; and both definitive and palliative interventions are probable, in the sense that we cannot predict their outcome accurately in any given case, though we can do so on the average in many cases. Therefore, we have the means to develop the well-accepted principle that the probability of aggregate benefits must outweigh the probability of aggregate harm. Heaney goes on to suggest that health care professionals too often are trapped in an intention ethic that allows them to neglect that bad outcomes can even happen, simply because such outcomes are not intended and because the professionals are trying to do good. The fact that the aim is to help the patient seems to justify almost any course, which is, of course, classic denial.

In reexamining these issues, certainly the clarification of bad to worse outcomes needs to be qualified. Therefore, to some extent the purpose of interventions needs to be examined. Clearly maintenance and restoration of health and maintenance and restoration of functional and relational capacity must be considered in our central purposes.

Heaney concludes by saying that the new technology is a problem because it dazzles us in its own right. We are confused about our purposes of using it. We have failed to appreciate the inherently probabilistic nature of the positive and negative outcomes of our intensive interventions, and we concentrate instead only on the outcomes intended. Too often we are doing more harm than good. What the system needs as a solution, Heaney retorts, is a patient care manager:

> Someone who combines the roles of patient advocate, knowledgeable advisor, triage officer, and channel of access to the system and necessary information — someone to help patient and family choose wisely when they are unavoidably disabled both by the unbridgeable gulf between them and the health care professionals and by the anxiety always provoked by illness. What is needed is someone who knows the system, knows what technology can and cannot do, and yet can stand back from it far enough to have a reasonable perspective.

Nurses can and must fill this role. There are no other logical providers who can rationally and objectively fulfill this role.

The third strategy is to develop nursing technology to promote efficient use of nursing resources. Imagine the future when people will carry their medical history on a credit card. Computer-assisted clinical prescribing of interventions will be available, as will a national computerized system of patients records. Imagine electronic diagnosis at home: consumers checking their health status by pushing a button on their "health watch." Imagine cardiac bypass surgery declining by 75% because of plaque-buster drugs. Imagine quality assurance standards generated from computer knowledge bases that are integrated with patient records systems and that flag problem areas. Imagine that people will become their own primary care practitioners: Imagine a computer printout of things you need to know prior to your patients discharge or about your health promotion task of the day. Imagine automation and robotics reducing hospital staffing to two full-time equivalents per occupied bed or per critical care case in the home. This is precisely what developing *nursing* technology is all about. Nurses in selected areas need to be responsible for the development of technology designed to improve the efficient delivery of nursing care.

We must begin imagining how systems can be developed with the "right" questions and answers that will help nursing find effectiveness and efficiency in its responsibilities, thus reducing the of hours charting, redundant communication follow-up and checking, and the redoing of work. It recently has been estimated at one medical center that 47 different points of contact are required in order to complete one patient's chest film.

Nursing informatics, artificial intelligence, computerized data, and information handling will provide key technology designed to improve resource efficiency for nursing. Nursing must not wait for others to develop this technology. One thing is clearly evident: As the demand for nursing continues to rise, we must learn to do things differently. It is hoped that by doing differently, nurses will be freed up to enhance and promote a caring environment, not just provide caring commodities. Without a caring environment, technology may not work (Benner, 1988).

Progress in technology does not correlate with advances in humanity. Technology is the way of the future — no one can argue that — but improvements to our humanistic makeup may or may not be the way of the future. Will we spend all our time, money, and effort creating a rational, technical, mechanistic system that services sufficiently and adequately a nation of dullards? We may be able to leave the speed and efficiency of gathering, exchanging, storing information and genetic DNA multiplication to high-tech corporations and to computer whizzes, but we had better take care to see that the substance of that information is not left to those same people.

Technology is not art, and information is not intelligence. For every computer genius, there ought to be another in the shadow, someone sitting back with mind and heart working overtime, making sure the human species maintains a little depth, a few resources, and a conscience. As we contemplate, in general, content-specific knowledge relative to undergraduate generalists and graduate specialists, I challenge you with the following: For every hour budgeted for technological training, match that hour with time for some reflective analysis of the human condition — history, art, poetry, philosophy, anthropology — all those experiences that make us aware of the possibilities of improving the species. In other words, take time to focus not simply on quantity or efficiency in our day-to-day, mechanistic, corporate-commodities decision world, but also on the quality of human life, which gives meaning, finally, to any decision that affects our future that directs our critical care actions in our day-to-day worlds.

Leadership is in each of us. It does not rest in the position of the person at the top. We must shirk our compulsion to perfectionism: "I can't move ahead unless I am absolutely sure I am right, and that I won't fall and get bruised." We must be willing to risk, and not just risk on the things that are a sure thing. We must quit seeking permission and approval. Get support but, not permission. Leaders-winners-nurses take chances. Like everyone else, they fear failing, but they refuse to let fear control them. Winners do not give up when life gets rough. They hang in until the going gets better. Winners are flexible. They realize there is more than one way, and they are willing to try others. Leaders-winners-nurses know they are not perfect. They respect their weaknesses while making the most of their strengths. Leaders fall, but they do not stay down. They stubbornly refuse to let a fall keep them from climbing. Leaders-winners-nurses do not blame fate for their failure, nor luck for their successes. They accept responsibility for their lives and are positive thinkers. They see good in all things. From the ordinary, they make the extraordinary. They believe in the path they have chosen even when it is hard, even when others cannot see the way. Winners are patient. They know a goal is only as worthy as the effort that is required to achieve it. Winners, leaders, nurses, make this world a better place to be.

References

Amara, R. (1988, November/December). Health care tomorrow. *The Futurist, 22,* 16-20.

Benner, P. (1988). *Nursing as a caring profession.* Working paper, American Academy of Nursing, Kansas City, MO.

Fuchs, V. R. (1968). The growing demand for medical care. *New England Journal of Medicine, 279,* 192.

Heaney, R. P. (1987). Human choices and the technological imperative: Values in conflict. In: *The Dean's Distinguished Lecture Series.* Philadelphia: University of Pennsylvania, School of Nursing.

Lindeman, C. A. (1988). *Nursing & technology: Moving into the 21st century.* Paper presented at the Conference on Food & Drug Administration, Annapolis, MD.

Searle, L. D. (1988). The extent of the nursing shortage in critical care. *Heart & Lung, 17*(6), 25A, 26A, 29A.

Wesbury, S. A., Jr. (1988, March/April). The future of health care: Changes and choices. *Nursing Economics, 6*(2), 59-62.

Response to Ryan: An Educator's Perspective

Clair E. Martin

The AACN 1987 position statement (American Association of Critical-Care Nurses, 1987) resolves that "AACN strongly recommends incorporation of critical care content and corresponding direct clinical experiences into baccalaureate nursing programs." The focus of this paper is the relative roles and responsibilities of both education and practice for the preparation of critical care nurses.

Nursing can and should incorporate critical care content and clinical experiences into the baccalaureate curriculum as an option for some students. The nature of the relationship between education and practice is an essential determinant of the efficient implementation of this goal.

It is appropriate that the profession explore the issues and seek consensus on this question. However, it is necessary to recognize that this question is not an isolated professional issue but is within the public interest. Dr. Ryan stated that projections indicate that 40% of all hospital beds will be critical care beds. I suspect that this is a conservative estimate and that it ignores that there have been and will continue to be substantial increases in community-based critical care. The public expectation is that nurses care for sick people. This expectation is fundamental to the social contract between the nursing profession and the larger society. Specifically, the public interest in an adequate supply of competent nursing care allows us considerable latitude in selecting students, designing curricula, and controlling entry and practice issues. Nursing has specific obligations and privileges under the social contract. Our inability or unwillingness to ensure that the public has adequate numbers of competent practitioners to provide safe care is a violation of the social contract and inevitably will result in increased external control and regulation of professional affairs. This will have a negative impact on both education and practice.

Nurses do not exist independently or in a vacuum. We must pursue responsible interdependent relationships if we are to make a serious response appropriate to a major health care profession. Although demand is not the only factor to be considered when making decisions about educational programs, it is nevertheless a significant factor. The AACN position statement is a responsible action consistent with the expectations of the social contract.

Dr. Ryan's presentation reflected considerable ambivalence about the technology component of critical care. I share that approach/avoidance ambivalence. However, her paper tended to lead to the conclusion that high tech is the essence of critical care nursing. Her three recommendations that (1) educational programs should focus on technology, (2) education and practice should constrain the use of technology, and (3) nursing technology be developed to promote efficient use of nursing resources support this conclusion.

The frequent equating of critical care with technology indicates one of the first responsibilities of education and practice: This is to make visible the *care* in critical care nursing. The context *is* high tech, but the essence of critical care nursing is the therapeutic use of oneself in relation to a vulnerable other's human responses in a life-threatening situation.

Relationship between Education and Practice

The first responsibility of both education and practice is attitudinal. Bridges must be constructed that connect practice and education. We are a practice discipline. We need each other if we are to meet our goals of excellence. Our primary emphasis does differ, that is, the principal goal of education is teaching and research, whereas the primary goal of practice is the delivery of care. For that reason, maintaining separate identities and policies is important. However, our overall goals are the same. This warrants implementation of a shared-value system that incorporates teaching. research, and administration with practice. The formulation and implementation of a single nursing culture is basic to excellence in both nursing education and nursing practice.

At Emory University, we are implementing a collaborative partnership between the nursing school and the nursing service. A partnership implies equal status of the participants. It implies interdependence. It implies a nonzero sum game context in which both participants win or both lose. It requires mutual respect, risk taking, vulnerability, and a willingness to reconsider some dearly held basic assumptions about each other and the way in which we relate and behave. The goal of the collaborative partnership is to become more than the sum of an excellent nursing school and an excellent nursing service. It is within this context of collaborative partnership that I believe the AACN position has the greatest opportunity for being implemented effectively.

Formulation and implementation of several demonstration projects are appropriate primary strategies for implementing the AACN resolution. Teachers and critical care clinical nurse specialists can identify the content and clinical learning experiences appropriate to the baccalaureate and master's level. This task would be facilitated by AACN identifying commonalities that transcend the critical care policies and procedures of individual critical care practice settings. A partnership between the teacher and clinical nurse specialist can provide the context within which efficient and effective student learning can be achieved.

The Nell Hodgson Woodruff School of Nursing has implemented a consortium to offer regularly a continuing education critical care program for nurses employed by the participating institutions. The curriculum is determined mutually and is implemented by faculty and staff members of the participating institutions. The process involved in this program could be a model for implementing the AACN recommendations.

The incorporation of critical care content and clinical experience in the undergraduate program will be costly. The faculty-to-student ratio necessary for this experience requires the exploration of alternatives. The use of staff nurses or graduate students as clinical preceptors is one option. The development of simulated learning experiences is also promising as a way to increase the students' clinical judgment in a safe, cost-effective way. In any case, the cost of implementing this proposal is a significant factor that should be shared by both education and practice.

Structure of the Undergraduate Curriculum

Let us assume a consensus that the undergraduate curriculum is to be expanded to include content and clinical experience in critical care nursing. The most casual observer will see that this curriculum looks like an inner tube that already has been patched so much that no space is available for an additional patch. We are challenged to ensure that graduates from nursing school reflect the common understandings and abilities expected of any college-educated person. In addition, the challenge to prepare generalists who can enter the nursing job market with a minimal disruption to the nursing service is increasingly difficult because of the rapid expansion of knowledge and technology.

Our effort to be all things to all people has produced an undergraduate curricular structure that emphasizes the greatest variety of student experiences in different clinical facilities. Every few weeks, students are rotated to a new clinical setting, generally with a new faculty member. This has resulted in undergraduate education being a series of opportunities for students to become oriented to new facilities and to "psych out" the expectations of the new teacher. They have limited opportunities to develop the depth of understanding that is basic to clinical judgment. Our interest in implementing a fail-safe plan of study has produced a consequence not unlike the human tragedies illustrated in Greek mythology. The thing that we seek to avoid we actually ensure occurring by our single-minded focus. We put all the bits and pieces that we think a student might need to know into the curriculum in order to avoid an error that reflects poorly on us.

There is no room to add critical care to the curriculum, at least not by tinkering with the curriculum and adding a patch. However, perhaps we could structure undergraduate education in a different way. Perhaps we could teach less, so students could learn more. This AACN proposal may be the catalyst that encourages us to redesign undergraduate nursing education.

An undergraduate curriculum that begins with an orientation to how professionals do nursing could provide a foundation for cafeteria-style offering of courses that allows the student to acquire some depth of understanding and ability in a chosen area. The generalist nurse prepared at the undergraduate level is retained in this proposal because the emphasis is on the process of providing professional care for the individual, family, and community.

A curriculum that promotes depth of understanding within selected settings should include the opportunity for students to compare and contrast the commonalities and differences of their experiences with those of students in other settings. The vicarious learning ability of students is exceptional within the informal system. Structuring this opportunity can amplify learning effects. The ability to transfer learning from one situation to another is enhanced.

Relative Roles of Students and Teachers

A new teacher-student relationship is an integral part of this restructured educational experience. The teacher at any point may have primary responsibilities for practice. The socialization studies of students reveal their identification with the "real" nurse as one who is practicing. The student's learning is the primary value in this restructured educational experience. The student is empowered as an active participant in the teaching-learning process. The traditional, rigid, hierarchical stratification of teacher-student roles is not appropriate for the typical contemporary student. Diekelmann (1988) uses the descriptive terminology of students on strike to illustrate the disengagement of students who are burned out and fed up with the passive role ascribed to them. Our students are bright. We need to free them to learn.

Introduction of critical care content and experience at the undergraduate level is possible and appropriate. Alternative strategies for meeting the increased demand for critical care nurses should be considered. An additional opportunity to provide adequate numbers of critical care nurses could be found in the programs being designed for students who hold a nonnursing degree. Our society will increasingly generate second career decisions. This means that individuals who bring life experiences appropriate to professional decision making can, after completing a "bridge" curriculum, successfully enter and complete the traditional graduate specialties.

Summary

The profession must respond to the demand for critical care nurses. One option that holds promise is the incorporation of critical care content and clinical experiences into the baccalaureate curriculum. Efficient implementation of this option requires consideration of the basic relationship between education and practice, the structure of the undergraduate curriculum, and the relative roles of teacher and student. This option provides an opportunity for nursing to clarify the essential care component of critical care nursing and the ethical dilemmas confronted by nurses in the provision of care.

References

American Association of Critical-Care Nurses. (1987). *Need for critical care content and clinical experiences in baccalaureate nursing curricula.* (AACN position statement). Newport Beach, CA: Author.

Diekelmann, N.(1988). Curriculum revolution: A theoretical and philosophical mandate for change. In *Curriculum revolution: Mandate for change.* New York: National League for Nursing. (pp. 137-158).

Response to Ryan: A Nursing Administrator's Perspective

Mary F. Woody

The subject of this conference and Dr. Ryan's paper, stirred a desire in me to search out and recall what our education and practice have been in the past in what we call critical care today. A brief summary reveals (Hilberman, 1975) that the placement of patients was the first practice model. In 1893, Florence Nightingale recalled the placement of patients in a small room leading from the operating theater. Patients remained there until they had recovered from the immediate effects of the operation. In 1923, a three-bed intensive care unit was opened at the Johns Hopkins Hospital for the postoperative care of neurosurgical patients. In 1930, a combined recovery room and intensive care unit was designed and built as part of a German surgical hospital. During World War II, intensive care facilities and trauma units were developed in Europe.

The impetus for the opening of recovery rooms in the United States was an effect of the domestic nursing shortage created by World War II. Recovery rooms were opened in operating rooms not being used at the Mayo Clinic in Rochester, Minnesota and the Strong Memorial Hospital, Rochester, New York, in 1942 and at the New York Hospital in 1944. In 1947, the Oschner Clinic in New Orleans opened a large recovery room. This unit was designed so that patients who had had new and complicated operative procedures could be kept for three days after surgery. Dr. Oschner stressed that nurses specially trained in an enlarged role were needed to understand the potential complications of surgery and the therapies available. The Millard Fillmore Hospital in Buffalo, New York, established an obstetrical recovery room in September 1945. Because of early detection and treatment of postpartum hemorrhage in this setting, a highly significant decrease in maternal mortality occurred.

Other strategies used by hospitals in caring for critically ill patients involved placing these patients adjacent to the nursing station. Private duty nurses frequently were employed by families to care for patients whose needs were beyond what the general nursing staff could provide. At times, this extended into group nursing in which two to three patients would have one private duty nurse. Physicians became aware that the skill and expertise of individual nurses doing private duty correlated with the prognosis of the nurses' patients. These nurses then were requested routinely by physicians to care for patients who had had specific procedures or had problems. (Hilberman, 1975).

In the 1960s, I was involved in establishing critical care units within an existing acute care hospital. The units were developed to bring together resources in response to the rapid increase in knowledge and technology. The bringing together of resources was to consolidate technology and supplies and, more importantly, to bring together the needed personnel. Even though the nursing service was involved intimately in the development of the unit, most of the education needed by professional nurses was provided by the medical staff. Nursing education did not embrace critical care because such care was perceived to be based on the medical model and would result in nurses nursing technology instead of patients. I venture to guess that had nursing service and education behaved in a more professional mode during those developmental times, we would not be having this discussion today.

Critical Care and Technology

Critical care is a part of our real world. I do not discount the need for health promotion or a focus on wellness; however, when a person requires repair of a brain aneurysm or treatment for acute liver failure, the care and therapy provided in a critical care unit is needed and wanted. Nursing must respond to the demands of society for excellent acute care and less to what nursing perceives that society needs. If nursing is unwilling to address society's demand for critical care, it will be done in some other fashion. In response to Dr. Ryan's question, "Does intensive care . . . decrease mortality and morbidity?", I do not have any hard data available at this time;

however, I do think that there is evidence that supports the claim that ICUs reduce mortality and morbidity.

Dr. Ryan has equated critical care with environments of intensive, complex, and sophisticated technology. On the basis of this equation, she has recommended major development of the baccalaureate curriculum in the area of technology, balanced with time for reflective analysis of the quality of human life. She also has suggested that our future educational endeavors should be guided by our technological practice role and should include strategies for keeping up with, constraining, and developing technology. She has challenged education to find mechanisms to keep nurses informed of new technological devices. Training in advanced technology is important, but we need to develop the wisdom to use and manage technology, to be able to drive technology so that it does not drive us.

Technology is a part of critical care nursing practice, but the focus of that practice is the patient. The critical care setting is an excellent environment for learning for baccalaureate students, not because they will see the latest monitor or infusion device, but because they will have increased exposure to patients' responses to care and an intense view of why nurses do what they do in response to patients' needs. Even though students can experience patients' responses to nursing care outside the critical care environment, the probability and intensity of the exposure are enhanced greatly within this setting. In line with Benner's work (Benner, 1984), if persons are exposed to normal or marginal experiences, they will need repetitive exposures to the experience in order to learn. In contrast, if a person is exposed to an extraordinary experience, a single exposure can result in learning. What better arena for learning than exposure to the extraordinary experiences available within critical care?

Redirection and Collaboration

Now is the time for nursing service and education to behave in a more professional mode. I think there will never be enough faculty members to be teachers of both theory and practice. In addition, large numbers of nurses in acute care settings have an expertise that has come about through day-to-day practice and learning in a rapidly changing environment. Therefore, these expert practicing nurses not only are the logical teachers of future nurse professionals but also are the better teachers. Growth of the profession of nursing will be stunted if we do not find a way for nursing service and education to work together in support of each other. Education and service must recognize and applaud the contributions each gives to developing our future generation. At the same time, nursing must accept the limitations inherent from working solely in the academic or the practice arena.

I think that the role of nursing service and education in teaching critical care nursing is to redirect the environment for the integration of education and practice. The integration of education and practice can be accomplished only by developing and instilling a willingness and desire to work together toward a common goal, a desire to collaborate for the effective delivery of quality patient care and the development of professional practice. This redirection requires that nursing service and education move toward a culture in which collaboration is inherent. An environment that is supportive of a collaborative model will create a culture in which nurses, through increased exposure and involvement in that environment, will enhance their perceptions of themselves, their practice, and their profession.

By drawing on the assets that are available from practitioners within the acute care setting and educators within the academic setting, a new climate can be created between nursing practice and nursing education. By using the combined strengths of the individuals and groups to the fullest, a closer and more productive collaboration of nurses with nurses will result. Nurses who are a part of a collaborative environment will share their knowledge with their colleagues. In time, each nurse will accept teaching and learning to be as much a part of their practice of nursing as delivering care and teaching patients.

Redirecting the environment through the integration of nursing education and practice will result in positive outcomes for individual nurses, nursing services, nursing students, schools of nursing, and the profession. An environment that encompasses the melding of nursing education and practice will help to do the following:

- Increase individual satisfaction with nursing as a career choice.
- Reduce the cultural lag between nursing education and nursing practice.
- Recognize and support the education of future nurses as part of the professional nurse's role.
- Increase the "goodness of fit" between nursing education's theory and clinical curriculum and the realities of practice.
- Support the education of nurses as part of the mission of acute care hospitals.

- Use all nursing resources optimally to increase productivity and to be cost-effective for schools of nursing and hospital nursing services.
- Ensure an adequate, long-run supply of nurses who are prepared appropriately for the realities of nursing practice and the future.

Summary

Incorporation of critical care nursing at the baccalaureate level does not necessarily mean lengthening or revamping an already packed curriculum. Critical care is an environment in which concepts already included in the present curriculum are exaggerated and occur frequently. The students' exposure to the extraordinary patient experiences available within critical care will result in meaningful learning. Technology is part of the practice realm, and teaching about its use needs to remain at the bedside. The frequency of technological change requires day-to-day practice to maintain expertise. Critical care will expose students to the use of technology, but mastery of how to use each technological device occurs during life-long practice as a professional nurse.

My objective as a nurse administrator in encouraging critical care nursing at the baccalaureate level is not to employ graduate nurses in critical care. On the contrary, I do not think that the critical care setting is the appropriate beginning for most novice practitioners. My objective is to make it possible for students to be exposed to a wonderful education and learning experience. For this objective to be accomplished, nursing service and education must create a collaborative environment in which combined strengths are used and recognized for their contribution to the development of our future nursing generation.

References
Benner, P. (1984). *From novice to expert: Excellence and power in clinical nursing practice.* Menlo Park, CA: Addison-Wesley.

Hilberman, M. (1975). The evolution of intensive care units. *Critical Care Medicine, 3*(4), 159-165.

SECTION 4
Conclusion and Summaries

Concluding Remarks

Marguerite Kinney

This conference has brought together a variety of points of view, and we are grateful for the willingness of all the participants to lend their expertise and ideas to this important task. In trying to summarize the many view expressed by both presenters and participants, several conclusions seem evident. first, there is not unanimity on the position of integrating critical care into the baccalaureate curriculum. However, there does seem to be a "hospitality of the mind" relative to the contributions critical care nursing can make to the education of a professional nurse. The recommendations and strategies also showed evidence of creativity and vision about how we can improve on what we are doing to prepare a professional nurse to practice in today's world.

Many useful recommendations have been made by the small groups and offered by our speakers. The following seem to be those on which the consensus is greatest:

- A cohesive package of existing AACN documents would bring together the resources for curricular decisions.

- Videotapes, interactive disks, and other learning aids are needed to support the teaching of critical care.

- AACN should form coalitions to develop support for how to teach in the clinical setting.

- Faculty and service professionals should work together to support student learning and nursing practice in the critical care environment; there is a great need for collaborative models.
- AACN members should become involved at the local level in these mutual, collaborative activities, participating as preceptors and mentors and in curriculum discussions.
- We all must work to get the word out, to discuss with colleagues in local and regional forums the issues identified here. It would be useful to publish in educational journals, rather than only in critical care journals.
- Interest was expressed in exploring post-baccalaureate models for preparing nurses for critical care practice.
- AACN should identify organizational models to facilitate collaboration between nurses in educational practice.
- We need to analyze further the data from the NLN survey to learn more about what is happening currently in schools of nursing.
- AACN also should consider collecting additional data on existing programs that integrate critical care and should publish these findings, including the outcomes of such programs.
- Exemplars of collaborative models also would be useful material to have available.
- AACN must extend the publics to which it relates in addressing these concerns, relating to such groups as deans and directors of schools of nursing, hospital nurse executives, and faculty groups.
- Hospitals should offer summer externships and work-study options as a way of supporting the provision of critical care experience for students.

These are only some of the many ideas that you have generated in the past two days. We thank you for the investment of your time and energies in helping to examine this complex issue and look forward to continuing dialogue.

Summary Reports from Triads

The following is a summary of the responses given to a questionnaire administered at the end of the conference to each triad of dean, critical care faculty member, and nursing service representative.

1. Please indicate the type of educational triad that you represent.

    Health science center   7
    Public institution   13
    Private institution   8

2. Is your triad in agreement with the AACN position statements?

    Yes   16
    No   0
    Somewhat   8

    Comments:
    - Agree with intent.
    - There is a need for further explication and definitions:
        - Critical care nursing
        - Critical care content — how much, placement in the curriculum
        - Meaning of "essential"

- Critical care skills
- Desired outcomes
- Believe it is impossible to rate yes or no. We do support the idea, but feel the content of critical care nursing needs to be defined.
- Position statement refers to direct clinical experience, not just integration of content or application of content. At issue is whether all students should or could have direct clinical experience.
- Agree with concept of collaborative approach to provide critical care content to undergraduates.
- Philosophically — will work towards implementation. Plan to include faculty and a variety of service agencies in future dialogue.
- Roles of service and education should be defined in preparation for collaboration.
- Aspects of it require much more discussion at our institution; ways to implement it, to implement it in how much depth?
- Implications need to be clarified further. We believe critical care nursing is built on a base of clinical nursing knowledge, advanced nursing clinical decision making. We believe we can do more to prepare students for complex decision making without specifically preparing for entry directly into critical care.
- Basically, we are in agreement. We have incorporated critical care concepts since 1973. As a senior experience, it is associated with leadership course 5 hours. Expectation regarding critical care credentialing and expertise is unrealistic for faculty. Please rethink.
- Extensive clinical experience *should* (may be) an option for some students. *All* students have some care content in telemetry.
- In agreement with teaching the essential content (also that content not taught must be identified). Also in agreement with experience in the critical care setting. This model is currently in practice in our area.
- Agree with the notion that critical care content (in some form) is appropriate for generic baccalaureate students; however, must decide if it is medical-surgical content, or specialty content, or advanced content. Also, must take a position on critical care content for associate degree diploma nurses (differentiated).

- Clarification is needed on what is the critical care environment and where is critical care nursing practiced.
- Further discussion is needed regarding these issues:
  - Direct clinical experience versus integration of content
  - Do all students require critical care experience and content?
  - Is critical care medical-surgical content, specialty content, or advanced content?
  - Should critical care also be included in diploma and AD programs?

3. **In what way has the conference influenced your thinking about critical care content in baccalaureate nursing education?**

Comments:
- Explore additional experiences for enrichment in all courses to maximize student learning of critical care nursing.
- Implications for curriculum development in general.
- Has confirmed belief that critical care content should be afforded its place in the curriculum.
- Content underpinnings of critical care need to be more explicit.
- Supports current practice.
- More is being accomplished than we're given credit for — affirm, teaching elements now.
- Identify and emphasize by exposures to experiences components of critical care that are in existence.
- Raised consciousness.
- Increased sense of value of clinical *experience* in critical care.
- Observation *only* in critical care *not of* value.
- Critical thinking skills needed by students.
- Appreciation of critical care knowledge occurs in a variety of settings.
- Great divergence in thinking.
- Brainstorming about alternative curricular patterns.
- Not enough critical care faculty — needs development for program success.
- Reinforced collaboration between service and education.
- Clarify and differentiate content versus knowledge necessary to undergird content.
- Less focus on technology.
- Look at specific content and skills.

- Reexamine role and scope of practice of critical care nursing.
- Use critical care settings for a greater variety of learning activities.
- Increase competency in problem solving, assessment, clinical decision making and management of medical regimen.
- Increase use of simulation and computer-assisted instruction to increase competencies.
- Promotion of sharing of content and experiences at the conference.
- Expectations of new graduates need to be more clearly defined.
- Encourage more input from service side on undergraduate curriculum.
- Pursue this concept on a statewide basis.
- Encouraged us to continue pursuing practice — education models that are innovative and address the need to incorporate this content.
- AACN must share responsibility for critical care nursing development.
- Reevaluate current program in light of insights gained.
- Content must be included. Experience should be optional.

4. **What do you plan to do as a follow-up to this conference?**

   Comments:
   - Increase *agency* dialogue toward utilizing ICUs and critical care nurses as preceptors. (Consistent response among most triads)
   - Focus on preceptor role.
   - Investigate tangible preceptor reward.
   - Discuss the conference with faculty and curriculum committee.
   - Determine what is viewed as critical care and how to address in curriculum.
   - Share models from other programs with faculty.
   - Maintain network with members from conference.
   - Continue to foster knowledge synthesis with students.
   - Reexamine competencies.
   - Consideration will be made of how we are teaching "technology" for nursing assessment and therapeutics in the context of "caring".
   - Encourage faculty to participate in local AACN.
   - Present to joint meeting of education and hospital directors.

- Explore strategies and resources to *maintain* current programs: externship and special group experience.
- Extend externships to ICU.
- Leveling of acute care content in baccalaureate and master's programs.
- Increase teaching alternative strategies such as interactive television.
- Utilize hospital practitioners to evaluate current assessment course and learning lab.
- Present conference information to local AACN chapter.
- Involve practice people on curriculum committee.
- Share with representatives from other area programs.
- Involve students in discussions of this issue.
- Apply concepts from conference to our new critical care nursing course.
- Reconsider timing of critical care placement in curriculum.
- Research suggestions made.
- Place summary of conference in hospital newsletter.
- Evaluate graduate nurses competency level in critical care upon entry.
- Continue with critical care nursing content.
- Plans underway: 7-week, 40 hours per week, clinical with preceptor. Critical care can be chosen.
- Develop demonstration project illustrating education-practice-collaboration: (content and clinical experiences in critical care).
- Look at faculty joint appointments and staff adjunct positions.

Conference Summary

The invitational conference ended on a note of optimism and commitment. The group of educators, administrators, and nursing leaders clearly had applied themselves to the task at hand in the small-group sessions and had accomplished much in a limited time. In order to summarize the material generated by the small groups, major themes and issues are organized and presented under the framework of the four purposes of the conference.

Purposes 1 and 2

The first two purposes were (1) to examine issues surrounding the inclusion of critical care nursing content in the baccalaureate curriculum, and (2) to achieve consensus on the need to integrate critical care nursing into the baccalaureate curriculum.

RELATED THEMES, ISSUES, AND QUESTIONS

- The relationship between faculty and service is often a problem. Faculty members need to assume the role of mentor, colleague, resource, and team member with staff members.
- The purpose of basic education needs to be reexamined.

- Today's work place demands specialization. Should critical care nursing be a specialty that requires a master's degree?
- Clear identification is needed of the roles of staff and faculty members in relation to assignment of students.
- Increased acuity in hospitals has caused a shift back to schools of nursing to increase responsibilities for increased clinical experience. Is some of this the hospitals' responsibility?
- Agreement is needed on what the entry-level baccalaureate graduate should "look like." Abilities, skills, and concepts include the following:
  - humanistic focus
  - integration and synthesis of previous knowledge
  - beginning level clinical judgment
  - ability to set priorities
  - motivation to enhance own learning
  - ability to use nursing process
  - knowledge of basic physiologic concepts, such as acid-base balance
- Faculty members cannot spend time maintaining clinical expertise and still meet other university commitments
- Although the critical care area may be a good place to learn, it is not necessarily essential that every student have a critical care experience.
- Relative responsibilities of faculty and service are a major issue. *Faculty* responsibilities include:
  - teaching complex reasoning skills
  - teaching skills
  - teaching decision making and resource utilization
  - tailoring educational methods to individual experience and student needs
  - formalizing creative mechanisms for faculty and staff collaboration
  - hiring and using clinically expert faculty members for role modeling

  Service responsibilities include:
  - providing adequate support and resources for graduate nurses
  - hiring and using prepared expert nurses with master's degrees to develop staff

- tailoring orientation and continuing education to individual experiences and needs
- formalizing rewards for preceptors
- Is it the responsibility of faculty members or service personnel to be clinically expert role models?
- Different curricular models are needed for different kinds of institutions.
- Critical care content, essential content, and core content need to be defined.
- Discrepancies in salary are so great between faculty members and service personnel members that clinically expert faculty are leaving to work in the clinical area.
- An integrated plan is needed for movement from novice to expert, which would include science base, skills, technology, and practical applications. The framework must also include reference to postgraduate and practice setting educational programs.

Purposes 3 and 4

The last two purposes were (3) to achieve consensus on the education of nurses who care for critically ill patients and (4) to develop recommendations and strategies regarding the educational preparation of nurses in critical care nursing.

RELATED THEMES, ISSUES AND QUESTIONS

- An essentials document should be developed that spells out the content and components of critical care nursing needed at an entry level.
- AACN members actively should pursue influencing curricular decisions by doing the following:
  - being a preceptor to students
  - seeking out positions on curriculum committees
  - developing articles on this topic for educational journals
  - working on communication on the local level between faculty members and staff members
  - soliciting input and involvement of faculty members in AACN

- The AACN organization should assist the process by doing the following:
  - developing new teaching methods, such as interactive videos and computer-assisted instruction, to assist in the teaching of critical care content
  - reexamining the certification process to allow credit for time faculty members spend working with students
  - cosponsoring conferences between schools and critical care organizations regarding teaching strategies
  - providing materials, such as position statements and references, to all deans and chairs of curriculum committees
  - distributing the results of this conference to schools and hospitals
- Data should be collected and published on existing programs that integrate critical care and on collaborative models.
- Strategies for mentoring and simulation should be developed.
- Critical care nursing outcomes should be used as a framework for developing content to be taught.
- The beginning critical care nurse needs knowledge and skills in the following:
  - physical assessment
  - rationale for use of basic technologies
  - ethics
  - principles of fluid movement and electricity (physics)
  - pathophysiology
  - organizational skills
  - data synthesis
  - stress management
  - psychosocial considerations
- Options for advanced practice preparation should be considered.
- Differences in service and academic expectations of new graduates should be addressed.
- Summer externships should be offered for students in critical care. These could be designed as work-study elective.
- Clinical ladders should be developed that are based on the novice-to-expert continuum.
- Better use should be made of the clinical hours of students, reducing such things as changing facilities, changing faculty, having to learn new documentation requirements.

- Parallel appointments should be made of hospital representatives in schools and faculty members in hospitals.
- Educational resources (such as learning laboratories) should be shared between schools and hospitals.
- Critical knowledge is needed for critical care practice. It should be identified and used for curricular development.
- This group should be brought back together in one year for follow-up.
- Partnerships should be developed between clinical agencies and schools.
- Research should be done on topics that can assist in developing strategies, such as identification of types of individuals successful in critical care, impact of ethical dilemmas, factors influencing entry of and turnover in critical care nursing and effectiveness of teaching team modules.

SECTION 5
Appendixes

Appendix A
Survey of Critical Care Curriculum in Baccalaureate Programs in Nursing

You have been identified by your dean or director as the most knowledgeable faculty member about the baccalaureate curriculum in critical care nursing at your institution. This questionnaire is designed to provide the American Association of Critical–Care Nurses with information about the baccalaureate curriculum in critical care nursing, the quality of preparation as perceived by faculty involved in teaching that component of the curriculum, educational preparation and experience of the faculty who teach critical care nursing, and factors within your institution which either facilitate or impede the inclusion of critical care nursing in the undergraduate program. The questionnaire will take approximately twenty minutes to complete. We appreciate your assistance in providing this important information. Please respond by May 23, 1988. Please return the completed questionnaire in the postage–paid envelope to:

> National League for Nursing
> Research Division
> 10 Columbus Circle
> New York, N.Y. 10019–1350

DEFINITIONS

Critical Care Nursing is defined as that specialty within nursing which deals with human responses to life–threatening problems. The *critically ill patient* is one who is characterized by the presence of, or being at risk for developing, life–threatening problems. The critically ill patient requires constant intensive, multidisciplinary assessment and intervention in order to restore stability, prevent complications and achieve and maintain optimal responses. The critically ill patient can be distinguished from the acutely ill patient by his/her physiological instability and vulnerability. *Critical Care nursing curriculum* is aimed toward preparing nurses to care for the critically ill patient.

Reprinted from *American Association of Critical-Care Nurses and National League for Nursing* Critical Care Curriculum Survey.

PART I RESPONDENT INFORMATION

1. In what capacity are you completing this questionnaire? (*Check any that apply*)
   - Critical Care Nursing Faculty. . . . . ☐ 1
   - Coordinator of course/faculty responsible
     for critical care nursing content. . . . . ☐ 2
   - Member of curriculum committee. . . . . ☐ 3
   - Other (*please specify*)_____. . . . . ☐ 4

2. Please indicate your highest earned degree (*check one*)
   - Doctorate/Nursing. . . . . ☐ 1
   - Doctorate/Non–nursing. . . . . ☐ 2
   - Master's/Nursing. . . . . ☐ 3
   - Master's/Non–nursing. . . . . ☐ 4
   - Other (*specify*)_____. . . . . ☐ 5

3. Which of the following do you identify as your primary area of clinical specialization? (*Check one*)
   - Medical–Surgical Nursing. . . . ☐ 1   Psychiatric/Mental Health. . . . ☐ 4
   - Maternal–Child Nursing. . . . . . ☐ 2   Gerontological Nursing. . . . . . ☐ 5
   - Community Health Nursing. . . ☐ 3   Other (specify) _____ ☐ 6

4. Are you currently certified or have you ever been certified as a critical care nurse (CCRN) by the American Association of Critical–Care Nurses (AACN)? (*check one*)
   - No. . . . . ☐ 1
   - Yes, currently certified. . . . . . . ☐ 2
   - Yes, have been certified. . . . . . ☐ 3

5. Please indicate the number of years of experience you've had in direct care of the critically ill (*check one*):
   - None. ☐ 1   (*skip to page 3, Part III*)
   - 1 to 2 years. . . . . ☐ 2   (*go to question 6*)
   - 3 to 5 years. . . . . ☐ 3   (*go to question 6*)
   - More than 5 years. . . . . ☐ 4   (*go to question 6*)

6. Please indicate when you last practiced critical care nursing (*excluding clinical teaching with students*).
   - Currently practicing. . . . . ☐ 1
   - 1 to 2 years ago. . . . . ☐ 2
   - 3 to 5 years ago. . . . . ☐ 3
   - Over 5 years ago. . . . . ☐ 4

PART II INFORMATION ABOUT OTHER FACULTY

Please provide information on other faculty members involved in the clinical teaching of critical care nursing. If there are no other faculty members involved in clinical teaching of critical care nursing, please check here ☐, then skip to Question 15, PART III.

	HIGHEST EARNED CREDENTIAL	# OF FACULTY
7	Doctorate/Nursing.................................	_____
8	Doctorate/Non–nursing.............................	_____
9	Master's/Nursing..................................	_____
10	Master's/Non–nursing.............................	_____
11	Other *(specify)* _____	_____
12	Total faculty involved in critical care *(other than yourself)*................................	_____
13	How many of the above are certified (CCRN) by the American Association of Critical Care Nurses?...........	_____
14	How many have been involved in direct patient care of critical patients within the past five years *(excluding clinical teaching with students)*?	_____

PART III CRITICAL CARE PREPARATION AT THE BACCALAUREATE LEVEL

15   How is content in critical care nursing provided in your undergraduate program? *(Check only one)*.

      Not currently offered......... ☐ 1   *(Skip to page 5, Part IV)*
      As a separate course......... ☐ 2   *(Go on to question 16)*
      Included in other courses..... ☐ 3   *(Skip to page 4, question 25)*
      Both in separate course and in other courses............... ☐ 4   *(Go on to question 16)*

Questions 16 through 24 pertain to programs in which a separate course in critical care nursing is offered.

16   Is the course required?....... ☐ 1   Is the course elective?........ ☐ 2

17   How many credits is the separate course? *(complete one)*

      Semester hours.......... _____
      Quarter hours........... _____
      Other *(explain)*.......... _____   _____

18   In what year is this course offered?

      Junior .... ☐ 1
      Senior................... ☐ 2
      Both junior and senior........ ☐ 3

19 Does the course include clinical practice in a critical care unit?
    Yes ☐ 1   No ☐ 2   *(If No, skip to question 25, this page)*
20 How many hours per week? _____
21 How many weeks? _____
    Does the clinical practice include:
22 Observation?   Yes ☐ 1   No ☐ 2
23 Provision of Care?   Yes ☐ 1   No ☐ 2
24 What is the faculty/student ratio for the clinical instruction in the course?
    One faculty per _____ students

Go to page 5, Part IV

Questions 25 to 34 pertain to programs in which critical care nursing content is provided as a *part* of one or more courses.

25 In how many courses is critical care nursing content included?
    One ☐   Two ☐   Three or more ☐
26 In what year is (are) these courses offered?
    Junior . . . . ☐ 1
    Senior. . . . . ☐ 2
    Both junior and senior. . . . . ☐ 3
27 Does the course include clinical practice in a critical care unit?
    Yes ☐ 1   No ☐ 2 *(Skip to PART IV, this page)*
28 How many hours per week? _____
29 How many weeks? _____
    Does the clinical practice include:
30 Observation?   Yes ☐ 1   No ☐ 2
31 Provision of Care?   Yes ☐ 1   No ☐ 2
32 Is the faculty member responsible for supervision of students both in critical care *and* on another unit?
    Yes ☐ 1   No ☐ 2 Faculty member has responsibility for students only in critical care.
    If **Yes,** the faculty to student ratio is:
33 1 faculty member: _____ students in critical care and _____ students on another unit.
                          a   b
    If **No,** the faculty: student ratio is:
34 1 faculty member: _____ students in critical care.

PART IV. EVALUATION OF CRITICAL CARE CURRICULUM

Please indicate your general assessment of the current critical care curriculum of your institution by responding to the following statements *(circle appropriate response)*.

35 Time allotted to theory related to critical care nursing

    5   4   3   2   1   NA
    Adequate   Somewhat adequate   Inadequate   Not applicable

36 Depth of theory related to critical care nursing

    5   4   3   2   1   NA
    Adequate   Somewhat adequate   Inadequate   Not applicable

37 Time allotted to nursing students to gain experience providing care to the critically ill

    5   4   3   2   1   NA
    Adequate   Somewhat adequate   Inadequate   Not applicable

38 Availability of clinical learning experiences *(e.g. experience in critical care units)*

    5   4   3   2   1   NA
    Adequate   Somewhat adequate   Inadequate   Not applicable

39 Upon completion of critical care preparation available in the BSN program, students *(check one)*:

    Can care for critically ill patients independently. . . . . ☐ 1
    Require minimal additional orientation to the care of the critically ill. . . . . . . ☐ 2
    Need substantial additional orientation in the care of the critically ill. . . . . . . ☐ 3
    Not at all prepared to begin practice in the care of critically ill. . . . . ☐ 4

PART V. BARRIERS TO CRITICAL CARE NURSING IN THE BACCALAUREATE PROGRAM

The following items have been identified as possible barriers to the incorporation of critical care nursing in baccalaureate curricula. For each item, please indicate the extent to which this factor has influenced curriculum decisions.

IN GENERAL, THE FACULTY BELIEVE THAT CRITICAL CARE NURSING (CCN) SHOULD NOT BE TAUGHT AS A SEPARATE COURSE BECAUSE:

		Not a factor at our school			Very Important
40	CCN is a specialty and the goal of BSN curriculum is to prepare generalists.	0	1	2	3
41	Critically ill patients are too sick to be cared for by undergraduate students	0	1	2	3
42	CCN is too technological	0	1	2	3

		Not a factor at our school			Very Important
43	The curriculum design does not allow for inclusion of another course	0	1	2	3

IN GENERAL, IT IS DIFFICULT TO PLACE STUDENTS IN CRITICAL CARE UNITS FOR EXPERIENCE IN PROVIDING CARE TO CRITICALLY ILL PATIENTS BECAUSE:

		Not a factor at our school			Very Important
44	Agency policy does not allow students to provide care in the critical care units.	0	1	2	3
45	The agency requires a student to faculty ratio which cannot be achieved in our program.	0	1	2	3
46	Nursing staff will not/cannot serve as preceptors for undergraduate students in critical care units.	0	1	2	3
47	There are not enough critical care units in which all our students can obtain experience	0	1	2	3

IN GENERAL, THERE ARE NOT ENOUGH FACULTY PREPARED TO TEACH CRITICAL CARE NURSING BECAUSE:

		Not a factor at our school			Very Important
48	There is limited opportunity for practice	0	1	2	3
49	Clinical expertise is not as valued as other aspects of the faculty roles	0	1	2	3
50	We have difficulty recruiting critical care experts into faculty roles	0	1	2	3

51 Are there other barriers in your institution to incorporation of critical care nursing?

_____
_____
_____

52 What factors in your institution have served as a *facilitators* to the inclusion of critical care nursing content?

_____
_____
_____

Please return the completed questionnaire in the postage-paid envelope to:

**National League for Nursing
Research Division
10 Columbus Circle
New York, N.Y. 10019-1350**

Thank you for your assistance.

Appendix B
Critical Care Nursing in Baccalaureate Programs

Christine A. Tanner
Jeanette Hartshorn
Peri Rosenfeld

Critical care nursing began to emerge as a specialty in the 1970s. At that time, coronary care units and intensive care units were few in number. Today, nearly all hospitals have critical care units. The education of the nurses who work in these units was, at first, "on the job" or provided through continuing education courses. Since those early days, the body of knowledge and research base in CCN has grown. Despite this growth, there is limited evidence of the inclusion of content specific to critical care in baccalaureate programs. Most of the data available are anecdotal and provide only examples of how this content is included in the curricula of some undergraduate programs. Experiences in offering elective or required courses in critical care have been reported by several authors (Clochesy, 1983; Geels, 1974; Mathew & Goodwin, 1983; Millen & Hufschmidt, 1984).

In 1984, the AACN identified inclusion of critical care content in undergraduate programs as a major area of focus. A position statement released that year entitled "Integration of Critical Care Nursing Concepts and Clinical Experiences into Professional Nursing Programs" outlined a number of steps that should be used to accomplish the integration of concepts. Specifically, the statement documents the need for students in consultation with faculty members and critical care practitioners, to utilize the nursing process in caring for the critically ill and their families. The statement confirms the need for appropriately prepared faculty (in both education and experience) to work with students. All of these changes should also be supported by a closer working relationship between faculty and staff.

Three years later, a position statement specifically outlined a mandate for inclusion of critical care content in baccalaureate programs. "Integration of Critical Care Nursing Concepts and Clinical Experiences Into Professional Nursing Programs" specifically notes the importance of including direct clinical experience in the care of the critically ill. The statement further recommends that the AACN "...in conjunction with baccalaureate schools of nursing and appropriate accrediting bodies" progress toward "...the development, implementation and evaluation of strategies to incorporate critical care content and direct clinical experiences in baccalaureate nursing curricula" (AACN, 1987).

The need for action directed toward CCN baccalaureate education was highlighted further by a study of critical care nurse supply and requirements, conducted by Levine and Associates for AACN in 1988. The study indicated a current "severe" shortage of critical care nurses, citing a 13.8% vacancy rate nationwide. The study further indicated that the current supply would have to be increased by 42% to 90% to meet the demand for critical care nurses in 1990; the shortage of baccalaureate and master's prepared nurses is even more acute, particularly in light of the need for "specialized experience and knowledge" and the ever increasing acuity of critically ill patients. Among the conclusions drawn from the study was the following:

> Although critical care requires considerable knowledge beyond basic nursing education, knowledge that according to survey respondents was not imparted in basic programs, there appears to be little educational involvement beyond brief episodic continuing education programs. Higher education in critical care nursing is a relatively untapped area that promises great potential for improving the quality of care received by critical care patients. (AACN, 1988, p. 11)

Although education in critical care nursing is only one of many avenues to resolution of the nursing shortage in critical care areas, it is nevertheless an important one. There are currently no data on the extent to which critical care nursing is already included in baccalaureate curricula, and little data on factors that facilitate or discourage its inclusion (Dunbar, 1986). The current study is designed to describe the current status of CCN education in baccalaureate nursing programs. The following questions guided this study:

1. To what extent are CCN content and experiences included in baccalaureate nursing programs?
2. What are the characteristics of CCN curricula at the baccalaureate level, in terms of the nature of the courses and the amount of clinical experience?
3. What are the characteristics (educational preparation, CCN experience, and CCN certification) of faculty responsible for teaching CCN?
4. What is the quality of the critical care curriculum and the level of preparation of the graduates as perceived by faculty involved in critical care instruction?
5. What are the perceived barriers to incorporation of critical care content in the baccalaureate curriculum?
6. What are the relationships among the faculty characteristics, perceived barriers, nature and quantity of CCN course offerings, and perceived quality of the critical care curriculum?

Methods

Data on critical care nursing education were collected in the summer and fall of 1988 through a survey questionnaire sent to all 455 basic baccalaureate programs in the United States. Survey methodology was the most appropriate because it served two important functions. First, it was necessary to collect data from basic baccalaureate nursing programs (e.g., number of faculty, number of clinical hours) to understand the current status of CCN in the nation's undergraduate programs. In addition, in order to identify need for change, some initial measures were needed to evaluate the perceived quality of the current CCN curricula and to assess obstacles in developing and implementing such curricula.

Questionnaire

The questionnaire was developed by the investigators for this study. One investigator and members of the AACN Task Force prepared an initial draft; it was reviewed by six individuals knowledgeable about CCN education and practice. The final instrument consisted of five sections:

(1) respondent information; (2) information about faculty responsible for clinical teaching in CCN; (3) critical care preparation at the baccalaureate level, including (a) the form in which CCN content and experiences were offered (separate course, or included in other courses); (b) the credit hours and contact hours in clinical practice; (c) the nature of clinical experiences (observation or provision of care); and (d) student-faculty ratio; (4) evaluation of the CCN curriculum, including the faculty's perception of new graduates' ability to practice CCN; and (5) perceived barriers to the inclusion of CCN in the baccalaureate program.

Scale scores were derived for two variables: evaluation of the CCN curriculum and perceived barriers to inclusion of CCN content. Evaluation of the CCN curriculum was comprised of two subscales: (1) the faculty perception of the new graduates' ability to practice CCN was a single item, rated on 4 points from "not at all prepared to begin practice in the care of the critically ill" to "can care for critically ill patients independently'; and (2) evaluation of theory and clinical experiences was comprised of the total score on four items, each rated on a 5-point scale, from adequate to inadequate. Internal consistency reliability for this 4-item scale was .89.

The perceived barriers scale was comprised of three subscales: (1) barriers due to faculty beliefs was comprised of four items representing views of the total faculty might prevent or discourage the inclusion of CCN in the curriculum; (2) barriers related to clinical agency policy contained four items representing the adequacy and availability of clinical facilities for CCN experiences; and (3) barriers related to faculty preparation was comprised of three items related to the clinical expertise of the faculty in CCN. Each of these 11 items on the barrier scale was rated on a 4-point scale of importance in influencing curriculum decisions, from "not a factor at our school" to "very important." Coefficient alphas for the three subscale scores were respectively, .68, .74, and .65; for the total scale, the coefficient alpha was satisfactory at .75.

Sample

In order to reflect the most comprehensive portrayal of baccalaureate nursing education, the survey was sent to the entire universe of basic baccalaureate programs in the United States. The data base at the National League for Nursing (NLN) was used to identify the 455 state-approved baccalaureate nursing programs. The survey was addressed to the director/dean of the program, with the request that the survey be sent to the faculty member most familiar with critical care nursing. Two mailings yielded a response rate of 85%. Responses were coded and entered by a critical care nurse who was interning at NLN's Division of Research. Open-ended questions were evaluated through content analysis.

Of the 385 respondents, 167 (43.5%) were directly involved in the CCN curriculum, either as a faculty member or as coordinator of the course that includes critical care nursing content. Of these, 29 (17.4%) held a doctorate as their highest degree, 142 (85%) declared medical-surgical nursing as their specialty, and 34 (20.4%) were currently certified in critical care nursing (CCRN), and an additional 12 (7.2%) had been certified at one time. This group of respondents was quite experienced in the care of the critically ill; 101 (60.5%) had more than 5 years of experience, and 41 (24.6%) had 3-5 years of experience. 59 (36.4%) are currently practicing while an additional 30 (18.5%)) have had experience within the last 1-2 years.

Results and Discussion

Inclusion of CCN in the baccalaureate curriculum: Of the 385 returned questionnaires, 371 contained usable responses to questions about the critical care curriculum. A surprisingly large percentage of programs offered some content on critical care nursing: 353 (95.2%). Ninety-three (25%) offered it as a separate course, 192 (51.5%) included it in other courses, and 69 (17.9%) included it both in a separate course and in other courses.

Nature of CCN Curriculum

Separate CCN courses: Of those 93 programs offering a separate CCN course, in 74 programs (80.4%) the course was required. For programs on a semester system (78), the range of credit hours was from 2 to 12, with mean of 5.5. For programs on a quarter system (9), the range of credit hours was from 2 to 9, with a mean of 4.67. In most instances, the course was offered in the senior year (87%) or in both the junior and senior years (7%). It includes a clinical component (95%) with opportunities for providing care (95% of those with a clinical component). The total number of clinical hours ranged from 6 hours to 272 hours. The average number of clinical hours was 103, with a standard deviation of 52.

The faculty to student ratio for these separate courses with a clinical component ranged from one to one to one to 12. The mean

Table 1: *Mean, Standard Deviation and Proportion of Respondents Identifying Barriers to CCN in the Baccalaureate Curriculum*

FACTOR	Mean	SD	Percentage
Faculty beliefs that:			
CCN is a specialty and the goal of BSN curriculum is to prepare specialists	2.06	1.08	69.3*
Critically ill patients are too sick to be cared for by undergraduate students	1.09	0.97	32.8
CCN is too technological	0.98	0.98	27.0
Curriculum design does not allow inclusion of another course	1.63	1.31	53.6
Experiences limited because:			
Agency policy does not allow students to provide care in the critical care units	0.54	0.93	15.5
Agency requires a student-to-faculty ratio that cannot be achieved in our program	0.75	1.10	21.8
Nursing staff cannot serve as preceptors for our undergraduate students	0.72	1.02	21.0
There are not enough critical care units in which our students can obtain experience	0.66	1.05	18.6
Faculty preparation is limited because:			
There is limited opportunity for practice	0.92	1.07	29.1
Clinical expertise is not as valued as other aspects of the faculty role	1.10	1.22	34.4
We have difficulty recruiting critical care experts into faculty roles	1.16	1.14	35.7

*Percentage of respondents who identified these factors as important or very important as barriers to CCN in the baccalaureate curriculum.

was one faculty to 7.5 students with a standard deviation of 2.3 students.

Both separate and integrated CCN courses: Two hundred and sixty-one (261) programs either included CCN in other courses or offered a separate course *and* included CCN in other courses. Respondents from 244 of these programs provided additional information. In 106 (43%), CCN content was included in only one course. In 98 (40%), it was included in two courses, while in 40 (16%), it was included in three or more courses.

Similar to programs with separate courses, programs offered integrated courses most frequently in the senior year (50%) or in both the junior and senior years (35%). Most (82%) included a clinical

Table 2. *Correlations Among Characteristics of CCN Courses, Barriers, and Quality of CCN Curriculum and New Graduate Preparation*

Quality	Barriers to Inclusion				Perceived	
	Total	FB	AP	FE	CCN Curr	Grad
Characteristics						
Nature of CCN	.15	−.18	−.04	−.07	−.15*	.08
Number of Hours	−.25*	−.25*	−.15	−.11	.40*	.24*
SF Ratio	−.10	−.04	−.06	−.11	.05	.08
N of Faculty	−.01	.12	−.12	.00	−.11	.10
Barriers						
Total	1.00	.8*	.61*	.68*	−.54*	−.15*
FB		1.00	.27*	.29*	−.32*	−.18*
AP			1.00	.14	−.43*	−.15*
FE				1.00	−.39*	−.05

*$p < .05$.

component with opportunities for providing care (90% of those that had a clinical component). The number of total clinical hours ranged from 2 to 270 with a mean of 66 hours and a standard deviation of 56. Clinical instruction was provided in one of two models: (1) the faculty member's only responsibility for supervision was for students in the critical care units (46%) or (2) faculty supervised students both in the critical care unit and on other units (54%). The average faculty-student ratio was about the same in both situations: one faculty member to every 7.6-7.8 students.

Characteristics of CCN Faculty

An average of nearly three faculty in each in each school were involved in CCN instruction. The reported range was 1 to 18. Approximately 25% of all faculty members teaching CCN had doctorates (13% in nursing, 12% in other fields). Approximately 25% of all faculty members reportedly were certified by the AACN (CCRN). The faculty members also reportedly had extensive experience, 65% had more than five years of experience in CCN practice.

Quality of CCN Curriculum

Respondents were asked to evaluate the adequacy of four areas of the CCN curriculum: (1) time allotted to CCN theory, (2) the depth of CCN theory, (3) time allotted to gain experience in CCN practice, and (4) availability of clinical learning experiences. A majority rated all of these aspects as "somewhat adequate" to "adequate." Time allotted to theory seemed to be a problem in 19.1% of the programs; depth of theory was judged to be less than adequate in 18.9% of the programs. Availability of clinical learning experiences is a problem in 17.3% of the programs. However, the time allotted for clinical experience is judged to be less than adequate by 31% of the respondents.

Nearly 1 in 10 (9.4%) of the respondents indicated that graduates of the BSN program were not at all prepared to begin practice in the care of the critically ill. A majority (232; 60.9%) felt that graduates would need substantial additional orientation to care for the critically ill. One hundred two (26.8%) of the respondents indicated that graduates would need minimal additional orientation to care for the critically ill, which only one felt that new graduates could care for critically ill patients independently.

Barriers to Incorporation of CCN in the Baccalaureate Curriculum

Respondents were asked to identify which factors adversely affected decisions about inclusion of CCN in the curriculum. The responses are summarized by item in Table 1. The items are rated on a 3-point scale, with zero not being a factor and 3 being a very important factor. The means indicate to some extent which factors stand out as the more important barriers; e.g., a mean of 2 would suggest that a factor is somewhat important in decisions about inclusion of CCN in the curriculum. In addition, Table 1 indicates the proportion of respondents who reported each factor as being either important or very important. Both analyses clearly show that faculty beliefs were the most important set of factors that create barriers to CCN in the baccalaureate curriculum. Of these, the belief that CCN is a specialty seems to figure most prominently.

The questionnaire also included two open-ended questions, asking respondents to identify additional barriers and facilitators to the inclusion of CCN in the baccalaureate curriculum. The responses related to barriers fell into eight categories: (1) not enough faculty with critical care expertise, (2) generalist orientation of undergraduate curriculum, (3) student-faculty ratio, (4) time limitations in the curriculum, (5) limitations in clinical agencies, (6) lack of texts written for beginning critical care practice, (7) lack of defined curricular content by NLN/ANA, and (8) lack of bachelor's prepared preceptors. Facilitators included the following: (1) faculty commitment, (2) acknowledgment of increased need for this area of practice, (3) students' interest and demand for ICU experiences, (4) good marketing for school, (5) demand for graduates to be prepared in ICU practice, (6) availability of clinical settings, (7) questions on state board exams, (8) use of certain models or theories, and (9) graduate programs in the school specific to critical care.

Relationships among the Characteristics of the CCN Courses, Barriers and Perceived Quality of the Critical Care Curriculum

To determine the extent to which relationships exist among selected characteristics of the CCN courses, the perceived degree of barriers, and the perceived quality of the CCN curriculum, Pearson's Product-Moment Correlation Coefficients were computed (Table 2).

Characteristics of CCN courses and faculty that were considered include: (1) nature of the curriculum measured on an ordinal scale (0 = not included, 1 = separate course, 2 = integrated in one or more additional courses, 3 = both integrated and separate courses); (2) total number of clinical hours; (3) the student-faculty ratio; and (4) the total number of faculty involved in teaching CCN. The barriers variables were the total barriers score, and the subscale scores on faculty beliefs (FB), agency policy(AP), and faculty experience(FE). The perceived quality was the overall evaluation of the CCN curriculum (CCN CURR) and the preparation of the graduate for practice in CCN (Grad). The only program characteristic that was related to perceived quality was the number of clinical hours. Whether CCN was included in a separate course, integrated, or in more than one course apparently had no relationship to the perceived quality. Also of interest is that the student-faculty ratio was unrelated to both perceived quality and barriers to inclusion.

Barriers to inclusion of CCN content are negatively related to the number of clinical hours. All other subscale scores on barriers were negatively related to the perceived quality of the program. In other words, the fewer the perceived barriers to inclusion of CCN, the higher the quality. These findings are not surprising.

Discussion

According to these survey results, a surprisingly large proportion of U.S. baccalaureate nursing programs include some critical care nursing content in their curricula. The faculty-student ratios tend to be low. The faculty involved in CCN education are well educated and quite experienced; nearly a quarter hold the doctoral degree and/or are certified in critical care nursing practice. Nearly two-thirds have more than 5 years of experience in CCN. Yet despite these results, there are several indication of the dilemmas that nurse educators face regarding inclusion of CCN content. These dilemmas are not unlike those related to inclusion of content in any other particular area of nursing practice. First, there apparently is little agreement in the profession about what constitutes generalist practice and therefore what would constitute educational preparation for such a practice. Nearly 70% of the respondents in this survey indicated that faculty in their school believed that CCN is a specialty, and this belief inhibited inclusion of CCN content. Faculty also believe that the curricula are already packed with content, and inclusion of additional specialized areas of practice is neither possible nor desirable.

Whether or not CCN is considered a specialty, its inclusion in the basic undergraduate curriculum may be directed toward several goals: (1) preparing for beginning level practice in a critical care setting; (2) acquiring greater confidence and skill in nursing practice that would be applicable in many settings, including technical skills (Mathew & Goodwin, 1983; Millen & Hufschmidt, 1984), use of nursing process and conceptual frameworks (Dunbar, 1986; Millen & Hufschmidt, 1984), increased organizational skills, communication skills with physicians, abilities in decision making (Mathew & Goodwin, 1983), and improved coping ability in stressful situations (Clochesy, 1983); and (3) pursuing postgraduate education in critical care by having early positive exposure to critical care settings. Respondents were not asked to identify which, if any, of these goals were the basis for the CCN education in their respective programs. However, the tremendous variability in the nature and amount of CCN in the undergraduate curriculum suggests that different goals may be operating.

If the goal is to prepare graduates for beginning level practice in CCN, these data suggest that the goal is not being realized. Sixty-one percent of the respondents felt that graduates of their programs would need substantial additional orientation to care for the critically ill. There is no agreement within the profession about which of these goals are desirable for "generalist" preparation, nor which are achievable within the context of baccalaureate education. The AACN 1987 position statement suggests that baccalaureate graduates need to have the "knowledge and skills to practice at an entry level in the care of patients with complex problems and needs," but it stops short of explicitly recommending that they be prepared for entry level positions in critical care units.

Another dilemma implied by these survey results is the relationship between education and practice, specifically, faculty involvement in clinical practice to maintain their own competency and practicing nurses' participation in undergraduate education. Nearly one-third of the respondents indicated that there is limited opportunity for their own practice; nearly one-fifth of the respondents indicated that nursing staff cannot serve as preceptors for undergraduate students. These figures, when taken together, raise serious issues about the possibilities for quality clinical education in CCN as part of the baccalaureate program.

The issues raised by prior research and by this survey were discussed at an invitational conference hosted by the AACN in March 1989. The goals of this conference were: (1) to examine issues surrounding the inclusion of CCN content into the baccalaureate curriculum, (2) to achieve consensus on the need to integrate critical care nursing content into the baccalaureate curriculum, (3) to achieve consensus on the preparation of nurses to care for critically ill patients, and (4) to develop recommendations and strategies regarding the educational preparation of nurses in CCN (proceedings from this conference are available from AACN, One Civic Plaza, Newport Beach, CA 92660). Participants in this conference included 120 nurses and nurse educators from 40 schools of nursing and associated clinical practice agency. Recommendations from the conference had been forwarded to the AACN Board of Directors for their action before this article went to press.

Conclusions

1. There is a tremendous variability in the nature and amount of CCN in the undergraduate curriculum. The amount of critical care content, the way in which it is offered, and the required amount of clinical time varies tremendously from program to program.
2. Faculty generally rate the quality of the CCN offerings as being adequate, although the majority indicate that clinical time is somewhat less than adequate.
3. The faculty indicate that graduates from most of these baccalaureate programs would need substantial additional orientation before beginning practice in CCN.

4. Nearly a quarter of the faculty involved in CCN instruction hold the doctoral degree and/or are certified. Nearly two-thirds have more than 5 years of experience in CCN.
5. Faculty report a wide variety of barriers to the inclusion of CCN in baccalaureate curricula. Both faculty beliefs about the place of CCN as a specialty and the role of baccalaureate education in the preparation of generalists, and requirements for low faculty to student ratios present barriers to nearly half the respondents.

In summary, there is a need to resolve several issues related to inclusion of CCN in the baccalaureate curriculum. These include: (1) the nature of specialist versus generalist preparation; (2) the goals for inclusion of CCN, (as well as content related to any other area of practice which may be considered specialized); (3) the relationship between education and practice, and the responsibilities of each in educating competent practitioners to provide safe care to critically ill patients.

AACN Recommendations

The AACN hosted an Invitational Conference on Critical Care Nursing in the Baccalaureate Curriculum in March 1989. Recommendations based on deliberations of the participants of that conference were forwarded to the AACN Board of Directors for their action. The following are recommendations approved by the AACN Board at their August 1989 meeting.

Actions of the American Association of Critical-Care Nurses Board of Directors Related to Critical Care Nursing in Undergraduate Education

In August 1989, the AACN Board of Directors approved the following actions:

1. To develop an essentials document that defines the essential competencies and content for differentiated levels of critical care nursing practice (associate, baccalaureate and graduate).
2. To develop and disseminate guidelines for roles of academic and service educators in the preparation of critical care practitioners.

3. To continue efforts to develop and disseminate educational resources to support the implementation of critical care content and experience in undergraduate and graduate programs.

References

American Association of Critical-Care Nurses. (1984). *Integration of critical nursing concepts and clinical experiences into professional nursing programs.* (AACN position statement). Newport Beach, CA: Author.

American Association of Critical-Care Nurses. (1987). *Need for critical care content and clinical experiences in baccalaureate nursing curricula.* (AACN position statement). Newport Beach, CA: Author.

American Association of Critical-Care Nurses. (1988). *Summary analysis of critical care nurse supply and demand.* Newport Beach, CA: Author.

Clochesy, J. M. (1983). Preparing senior nursing students through optional clinical experiences. *Dimensions of Critical Care Nursing, 2*(6), 366-370.

Dunbar, S. (1986). Imperatives for nursing education. *Heart & Lung, 15*(6), 18A-22A.

Geels, W. J., Brand, L. M., & Passos, J. Y. (1974). The ICU and collegiate nursing education. *Journal of Nursing Education, 13*(1), 15-20.

Mathew, D. M., & Goodwin, M. H. (1983). Critical care practicum. *Focus on Critical Care, 10*(1), 38-42.

Millen, D. L., & Hufschmidt, A. P. (1984). Preparing the undergraduate for critical care. *Dimensions of Critical Care Nursing, 3*(5), 307-312.

Acknowledgments and Author Information

Christine A. Tanner, PhD, RN, FAAN, is professor of Adult Health and Illness Nursing, Oregon Health Sciences University School of Nursing, Portland, Oregon. She was chair of the AACN Invitational Conference Task Force on Critical Care Nursing Curriculum at the time this survey was conducted. Jeanette Hartshorn, PhD, RN, FAAN, is Associate Professor, College of Nursing, Medical University of South Carolina, Charleston South Carolina. She was immediate past president of AACN at the time this survey was conducted. Peri Rosenfeld, PhD is director, Research Division, National League for Nursing, New York, New York. The assistance of members of the Invitational Conference Task Force and the Education Special Interest Group in the design of the survey instrument is acknowledged. They are Kathleen Andreoli, Jan Boller, Barbara Daly, Sandra Goodnough, Marguerite Kinney, Mairead Hickey, and Chris Winkelman. Special acknowledgment to Jan Boller, Sandra Goodnough, and Linda Searle for their thoughtful comments on earlier versions of this article.

Appendix C
Getting Them Together

Molly Billingsley

To regular readers of this column, it must seem that I find problems under every professional rock. It really isn't my intention to chronically whimper and whine. It's just that a steady stream of things seems to cross my horizon at editorial time that cry out for some sort of comment. This month, a report came along that caught my attention for different reasons. I speak of the recent invitational conference sponsored by the American Association of Critical-Care Nurses (AACN) on integrating critical care into the baccalaureate curriculum. What made this conference different and refreshing is that the invited participants were deans, nursing faculty, nursing service administrators, and critical care nurses. At last a collaborative effort to work on a current nursing issue!

The conference grew out of a 1987 position paper from AACN's Education Special Interest Group (SIG). This statement, "Need for Critical Care Content and Clinical Experiences in Baccalaureate Nursing Curricula," was approved by the board. They also accepted the reality that a unilateral statement by a professional organization, even one as large and prestigious as AACN, was probably not going to provoke much movement in the greater scheme of things. Ergo, the unusual idea of bringing people together from the clinical area who have input on an idea and faculty and administration from nursing schools who have the power to implement the idea. Not only were they brought together to listen to speeches, they were

---

REPRINTED WITH PERMISSION FROM *NURSING CONNECTIONS* 2(2) (SUMMER 1989).

made to hash out differences in a small group format. This is an amazing step forward.

It was an opportunity for all who attended to broaden horizons. Doubtless a number of the "big name experts" who participated learned as much as anyone. There is nothing like a direct report from someone who actually works in the trenches to rock your theoretical boat. Insights were not limited to the heavily initialled, however. Critical care clinicians and administrators from big city hospitals, heavily are in favor of increasing critical care content in undergraduate studies, listened in amazement to a rural contingent who reported that the number of ICU beds in their entire area could be counted on both hands (and often went unfilled). Which is, of course, the point of the exercise. Nurses in education and practice have so firmly grasped their respective parochial versions of truth that both have lost sight of the fact that truth comes in many shades.

What were the final outcomes? Naturally, the first recommendation was to establish the obligatory task force to define the terms (nursing task avoidance strategy No. 1). Second, most participants agreed that schools probably could not do much more than provide the barest essentials of critical care nursing, particularly since one of the few things most of us agree on is that baccalaureate education prepares a generalist.

Finally, everyone did seem to agree that certain analytic skills and basic content such as cardiac dysrhythmias, bioethical decision making, and selected techniques of advanced physical assessment are vital in the undergraduate curriculum.

Nothing world-shattering, perhaps. I do not know whether the AACN was thrilled with the results. But I think it was auspicious. If all specialty groups (including the generalists, the biggest specialty group of all) looked at this model and convened such symposia on a regular basis, the gap between education and practice would rapidly become a thing of the past.

The editorial mission of *Nursing Connections* is to celebrate successful collaborative efforts. AACN, cheers!

Author Information
Molly Billingsly, RNC, MSN, EdD, is editor-in-chief of *Nursing Connections* and associate director of nursing at The Washington Hospital Center, Washington, DC.